Mayo Clinic on High Blood Pressure

Sheldon G. Sheps, M.D.

Editor in Chief

Mayo Clinic

Rochester, Minnesota

Mayo Clinic on High Blood Pressure provides reliable, practical, easy-to-understand information on preventing and managing high blood pressure. Much of the information comes directly from the experience of doctors, nurses, registered dietitians, health educators and other health care professionals at Mayo Clinic. This book supplements the advice of your personal physician, whom you should consult for individual medical problems. *Mayo Clinic on High Blood Pressure* does not endorse any company or product. MAYO, MAYO CLINIC, MAYO CLINIC HEALTH INFORMATION and the Mayo triple-shield logo are marks of Mayo Foundation for Medical Education and Research.

Published by Mayo Clinic Health Information, Rochester, Minn. Distributed to the book trade by Kensington Publishing Corporation, New York, NY.

Menu analysis was done by Mayo Clinic registered dietitians using Nutritionist IV software by N-Squared.

Library of Congress Catalog Card Number 2002113871

ISBN 1-893005-26-7

Printed in the United States of America

Second Edition

1 2 3 4 5 6 7 8 9 10

About High Blood Pressure

One in four adults in the United States has high blood pressure. You or a family member may be one of them.

High blood pressure is a deceptive illness because it causes few, if any, symptoms. That's why few people view it as a life-threatening condition. Nothing could be further from the truth. High blood pressure is a leading cause of stroke, heart attack, heart failure, kidney failure, dementia and premature death. If you don't take it seriously, it can shorten your life by 10 to 20 years.

There is no cure for high blood pressure. But the good news is the condition is both preventable and treatable. Adjustments to your lifestyle and, if necessary, medication can help you take control of your blood pressure and keep it at a safe level. This book offers practical advice you can put to use today to better manage your blood pressure. Much of the information is used daily by Mayo Clinic doctors and other health care professionals in caring for their patients.

About Mayo Clinic

Mayo Clinic evolved from the frontier practice of Dr. William Worrall Mayo and the partnership of his two sons, William J. and Charles H. Mayo, in the early 1900s. Pressed by the demands of their busy practice in Rochester, Minn., the Mayo brothers invited other physicians to join them, pioneering the private group practice of medicine. Today, with more than 2,000 physicians and scientists at its three major locations in Rochester, Minn., Jacksonville, Fla., and Scottsdale, Ariz., Mayo Clinic is dedicated to providing comprehensive diagnoses, accurate answers, and effective treatments.

With this depth of medical knowledge, experience and expertise, Mayo Clinic occupies an unparalleled position as a health information resource. Since 1983, Mayo Clinic has published reliable health information for millions of consumers through a variety of award-winning newsletters, books and online services. Revenue from these publishing activities supports Mayo Clinic programs, including medical education and medical research.

Editorial staff

Editor in Chief
Sheldon G. Sheps, M.D.

Managing Editor
Richard Dietman

Editorial Research
Anthony Cook
Danielle Gerberi
Deirdre Herman
Michelle Hewlett

Proofreading
Miranda Attlesey
Donna Hanson
Judith Shuster

Contributing Writers
Anne Christiansen
D.R. Martin
Stephen Miller
Doug Toft
Susan Wichmann

Creative Director
Daniel W. Brevick

Design
Craig King

Illustration and Photography
John Hagen
Michael King
Richard Madsen
Kent McDaniel
Christopher Srnka

Indexing
Larry Harrison

Contributing editors and reviewers

Tammy Adams, R.N.
Tracy Berg, R.Ph.
Brent Bauer, M.D.
Helmut Buettner, M.D.
Christopher Frye
Andrew Good, M.D.
John Graves, M.D.
Sharonne Hayes, M.D.
Donald Hensrud, M.D.
John E. Hodgson, L.P.
Richard Hurt, M.D.
Patricia Jensen, R.N.
Todd Johnson, Pharm.D.
Nancy Kaufman, R.D., M.P.H.
Keith Kramlinger, M.D.
Edward Laskowski, M.D.
Bruce Morgenstern, M.D.
Carol Nash, R.N.
Jennifer K. Nelson, R.D.
Sandra Taler, M.D.
Stephen Turner, M.D.
Beth Warren
Donald Williams, Ph.D.

Preface

The more you know about high blood pressure, the better prepared you'll be to take the necessary steps to lower your blood pressure and keep it under control. That was the focus of the first edition of *Mayo Clinic on High Blood Pressure* — published in 1999 and translated into nine languages — and it's the guiding principle behind this revised and updated second edition.

The past 40 years have brought major advances in identifying and treating high blood pressure. Greater attention to this common illness is a major reason deaths from stroke have decreased 70 percent and deaths from heart disease are down more than 56 percent.

Still, high blood pressure remains a serious problem. Of the 50 million Americans with the condition, 31 percent are unaware they have it and 17 percent are aware but not being treated. This is disturbing considering that high blood pressure can almost always be successfully managed.

In this new second edition, you'll learn how high blood pressure develops and why it's so harmful when it's not controlled. You'll also learn the steps you can take to reduce your risk of coronary artery disease, heart failure, kidney failure, stroke and dementia — all problems associated with high blood pressure. New information on insulin resistance syndrome, sleep apnea and herbal supplements has been added. And you'll find the latest on issues of concern to women, children, older adults and special at-risk populations, including those with diabetes. You'll also read about proper use of medications, monitoring your blood pressure at home and regular follow-up care.

Mayo Clinic doctors, nurses, registered dietitians, pharmacists, psychologists, researchers and health educators reviewed these chapters to ensure that you receive the latest and most accurate information. This book, along with the advice of your personal physician, can help you live a longer, healthier life.

Sheldon G. Sheps, M.D.
Editor in Chief

Contents

Chapter 1

What is high blood pressure?

If you're like many Americans, your blood pressure may be too high. That worries you, and that's why you're reading this book. Unfortunately, many people think that having high blood pressure isn't a big deal. It is. High blood pressure is one of the leading causes of disability or death due to stroke, heart attack, heart failure, kidney failure and dementia.

Consider the numbers

High blood pressure — also called hypertension — is the most common chronic illness in the United States. According to the National Heart, Lung, and Blood Institute (NHLBI), almost 50 million Americans have high blood pressure. That's about one out of every four adults. Each year, 2 million new cases of the disease are diagnosed. In the year 2000, high blood pressure accounted for almost 10.4 million visits to doctors' offices.

However, high blood pressure often isn't given the attention it deserves. Many people affected by high blood pressure don't even know they have it. A major reason is that the disease generally doesn't produce symptoms until it has progressed to an advanced stage. Of those with high blood pressure, about 68 percent are aware of their condition, but only 27 percent have it under control.

When it comes to controlling high blood pressure, a couple of factors complicate the picture. One is age. People can develop high blood pressure at any time, but the risk increases with age. According to a 2002 update of the NHLBI's landmark Framingham Heart Study, middle-aged Americans face a 90-percent chance of developing high blood pressure. And it's estimated that 60 percent of Americans age 65 and older have high blood pressure.

Another factor is race. About 23 percent of white Americans ages 18 to 74 have high blood pressure. Among blacks, the number jumps to about 33 percent. For American Indians, the number is 21 percent, for Hispanics it's 18 percent, and for Americans of Asian and Pacific Islander descent, it's 16 percent.

But there's also good news. High blood pressure doesn't have to be deadly or disabling. The condition is easy to detect. And among cardiovascular diseases, high blood pressure is the most treatable. Once you know you have high blood pressure, you can take steps to lower it to a safe level. Bringing your blood pressure down to the optimal range for 5 or more years greatly reduces your risk of cardiovascular diseases. The two main methods for treating high blood pressure are changes in your lifestyle and medication.

You can live long and live well after receiving a diagnosis of high blood pressure. But you have to be willing to do your part to keep your blood pressure under control. Whether your high blood pressure was recently diagnosed, you've had it for many years or you simply want to prevent it, this book can help you learn more about the disease. You'll also find out how your daily life affects your blood pressure and learn ways you can change bad habits into healthy ones.

The basics of blood pressure

To better control your blood pressure, it helps to know some basics about the role of blood pressure and the organs and systems that help to regulate it. This will make it easier to understand how high blood pressure develops and why it can be so harmful.

Your cardiovascular system

An understanding of blood pressure begins with your cardiovascular system, the system responsible for circulating blood through your heart and blood vessels (see illustration on page 4).

With each beat of your heart, a surge of blood is released from your heart's main pumping chamber (left ventricle) into an intricate web of blood vessels that spread throughout your body.

Your arteries are the blood vessels that carry nutrient- and oxygen-rich blood from your heart to your body's tissues and organs. The largest artery, called the aorta, is connected to the left ventricle and serves as the main channel for blood leaving your heart. The aorta branches off into smaller arteries, which turn into even smaller arteries, called arterioles.

Within your body's tissues and organs are microscopic blood vessels called capillaries. The capillaries exchange nutrients and fresh oxygen from the arterioles for carbon dioxide and other waste products produced by your cells. This oxygen-depleted blood is sent back to your heart through a system of blood vessels called veins.

When it reaches your heart, blood from your veins is routed to your lungs, where it releases carbon dioxide and picks up a new supply of oxygen. This freshly oxygenated blood is sent back to your heart, ready to begin another journey. Other waste products are removed as your blood passes through your kidneys and liver.

To keep this system working and all of the 11 pints of blood in your body moving, a certain amount of pressure is required. Your blood pressure is the force that's exerted on your artery walls as blood passes through. This force helps to keep blood in your arteries flowing smoothly.

Blood pressure is often compared to the pressure inside a garden hose. Without some type of force to push the water, it couldn't get from one end of the hose to the other.

Regulators of blood pressure

Several systems help control your blood pressure and keep it from rising too high or falling too low. They include your heart, arteries, kidneys, various hormones and enzymes, and your nervous system.

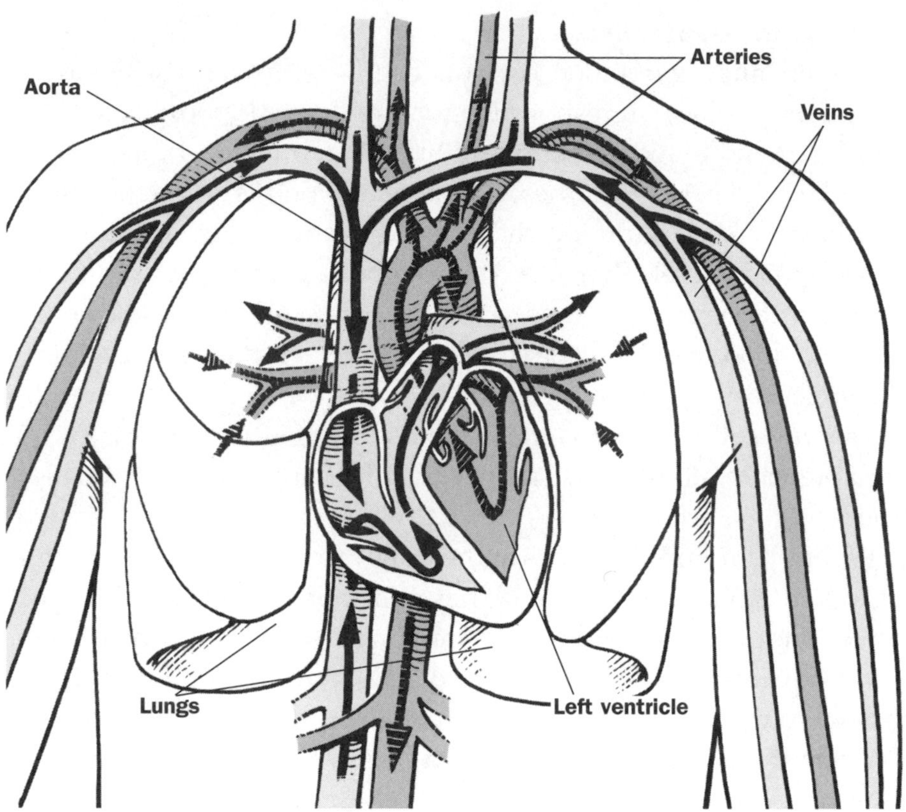

Each time your heart beats, blood is released from the left side of your heart (left ventricle) into the large blood vessel (aorta) that transports blood to your arteries. Blood returns to your heart through your veins. Before being circulated again, blood from your veins is sent to your lungs to load up on fresh oxygen.

Your heart. When your heart releases blood into your main artery (aorta), a certain amount of force is created by the pumping action of your heart muscle. The harder your heart muscle has to work to pump blood, the greater is the force exerted on your arteries.

Your arteries. To accommodate the surge of blood coming from your heart, your arteries are lined with smooth muscles that allow them to expand and contract as blood courses through. The more elastic your arteries are, the less resistant they are to the flow of blood, and therefore less force is exerted on their walls. When arteries lose their elasticity or they become narrowed, resistance to blood flow increases and additional force is needed to push blood through the vessels. This increased force can contribute to higher blood pressure.

Your kidneys. Your kidneys regulate the amount of sodium in your body and the volume of water circulating in your body. Sodium retains water. Therefore, the more sodium that's in your system, the more water that's contained in your blood. This extra fluid can increase blood pressure. In addition, too much sodium can cause your blood vessels to narrow.

Other factors. Your central nervous system, along with hormones, enzymes and other chemicals, also influences your blood pressure.

Baroreceptors. Within the walls of your heart and several blood vessels are tiny node-like structures called baroreceptors. These structures work similar to the thermostat in your house. Baroreceptors continuously monitor the pressure of blood in your arteries and veins. If they sense a change in pressure, they send signals to your brain to slow down or speed up your heart rate or to widen or narrow your arteries to keep your blood pressure within a normal range.

Epinephrine. Your brain acts on messages from the baroreceptors by signaling the release of hormones and enzymes that affect the functioning of your heart, blood vessels and kidneys. One of the most significant hormones to affect blood pressure is epinephrine (ep-ih-NEF-rin), also known as adrenaline. Epinephrine is released into your body during periods of high stress or tension, such as when you're frightened or hurrying to complete a task.

Epinephrine causes your arteries to narrow and your heart contractions to become stronger and more rapid, increasing pressure in your arteries. People often refer to the effect of epinephrine as feeling pumped up or on an adrenaline high. (See "The stress response" on page 133.)

The renin-angiotensin-aldosterone system. Researchers are studying the role of other hormones as well. These include renin (RE-nin), which your body converts into another hormone called angiotensin (an-je-o-TEN-sin) I . When it reaches your bloodstream, angiotensin I is converted into a substance called angiotensin II. In turn, angiotensin II constricts your blood vessels and stimulates release of a hormone called aldosterone (al-DOS-tur-own) from the adrenal gland. One result of increased aldosterone is that your kidneys retain more water and sodium.

Researchers believe that some people with high blood pressure have a variation in the gene that determines their body's release of angiotensin. As a result, the body produces too much of this hormone.

The endothelium. The walls of your arteries and veins have an extremely thin lining of cells. This lining is called the endothelium. Research has shown that the endothelium plays a crucial role in regulating blood pressure — for example, by secreting chemicals that cause blood vessels to contract and relax.

Nitric oxide. A gas called nitric oxide, which is present in your arteries and blood, can affect your blood pressure. This gas signals blood vessels to relax and expand. Nitroglycerin, a medication used to treat some forms of cardiovascular disease, increases levels of nitric oxide.

Endothelin. In contrast to nitric oxide, a protein called endothelin (en-do-THE-lin) acts as a potent vasoconstrictor. It causes blood vessels to narrow. Endothelin-1, one form of this protein, may play a crucial role in the development of high blood pressure.

What the numbers mean

Your blood pressure is determined by measuring the pressure within your arteries. This is done with an instrument called a sphygmomanometer (sfig-mo-muh-NOM-uh-tur). It includes an inflatable cuff that's wrapped around your upper arm, an air pump, and a standardized pressure gauge or a digital meter.

Blood pressure is expressed in terms of millimeters of mercury (mm Hg). The measurement refers to how high the pressure in your arteries is able to raise a column of mercury on the sphygmomanometer.

Two measurements

Two numbers are involved in a blood pressure reading. Both are equally important. The first of the two is your systolic (sis-TOL-ik) pressure. This is the amount of pressure in your arteries when your heart contracts — called systole (SIS-to-le) — and releases blood into the aorta. The second number is your diastolic (di-uh-STOL-ik) pressure. It tells how much pressure remains in your arteries between beats when your heart is relaxing — called diastole (di-AS-to-le) — and filling with blood. Your heart muscle must relax fully before it can contract again. During this time, your blood pressure decreases.

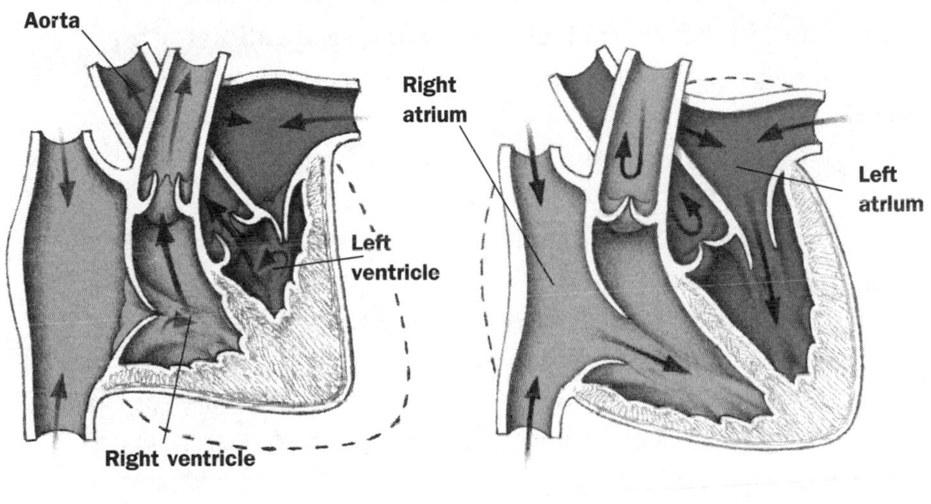

During systole (left), your heart muscle squeezes blood out of your heart's pumping chambers (ventricles). Blood on the right side of your heart goes to your lungs, and blood on the left side is pumped into the large blood vessel (aorta) that feeds your arteries. During diastole (right), your heart muscle relaxes and expands to allow blood to flow into the pumping chambers from your heart's holding chambers (atria).

The two numbers are usually written to look like a fraction. Systolic pressure is placed above or to the left and the diastolic pressure is placed below or to the right. When stated verbally, the word *over* is generally used to separate the two numbers. For example, if your systolic pressure is 115 mm Hg and your diastolic pressure is 82 mm Hg, you have a blood pressure of 115/82, or 115 over 82.

In the first few months after birth, a baby's blood pressure is around 100/65 mm Hg, or 100 over 65. During childhood, it slowly increases. In adulthood, the optimal range of blood pressure is 119/79 mm Hg or lower. The normal range is 129/84 mm Hg or lower. Systolic blood pressures between 130 and 139 mm Hg and diastolic pressures between 85 and 89 mm Hg are at the high end of what's considered a safe level. Readings within these ranges are referred to as high-normal. (See "Classification of blood pressure" on page 9.)

An ideal or optimal blood pressure for an adult of any age is 119/79 mm Hg or lower. This is what you should aim for, if possible. For certain individuals who are taking medication for high blood pressure, a blood pressure that low may not be reasonable or tolerable.

Daily ups and downs

A blood pressure reading reflects only what your blood pressure is at the moment it's measured. Throughout the day, your blood pressure naturally fluctuates. It increases during periods of activity when your heart has to work harder, such as when you exercise. And it decreases with rest when there's less demand on your heart, such as when you sleep. Your blood pressure also changes with changes in your body position, such as when you move from a lying or sitting position to a standing position. (See "When your blood pressure drops too low" on page 12.)

Food, alcohol, pain, stress and strong emotions also increase your blood pressure. Even while you sleep, dreaming can raise your blood pressure. These ups and downs are perfectly normal.

Your blood pressure even changes with the time of day. Pressure in your arteries follows a natural fluctuation during a 24-hour period. It's usually the highest in the morning hours after you awaken and become active. It generally stays at about the same level throughout the day and then late in the evening it begins to decrease. It reaches its lowest level in the early morning hours while you're sleeping. This 24-hour pattern is known as a circadian (sur-KAY-de-un) rhythm. Your body has more than 100 circadian rhythms, each influencing a different body function.

If you're an evening or overnight shift worker, the circadian rhythm of your blood pressure is different from that of a day worker and is more closely aligned to your schedule of work and rest. That's because many circadian rhythms change with altered patterns of activity.

Getting an accurate reading

To get a good indication of what your average blood pressure is, the best time to measure it is during the day after you've been active for a few hours. If you exercise in the morning, it's better to measure your blood pressure beforehand. After strenuous physical activity, your blood pressure may stay at a temporarily low level. Readings taken during this time may not reflect your average pressure.

You also shouldn't eat, smoke or drink caffeine or alcohol 30 minutes before measuring your blood pressure. Tobacco and caffeine can temporarily increase your pressure. Alcohol may temporarily decrease your blood pressure. In some people, though, alcohol has the opposite effect. It increases blood pressure. Some over-the-counter medications, including decongestants, anti-inflammatory drugs and certain diet aids, can increase your blood pressure for hours or even days after you take them. In addition, you should wait 5 minutes after you sit down before taking a reading so that your blood pressure has time to adjust to your change in position and activity. Measuring your blood pressure under these

Classification of blood pressure

	Systolic (mm Hg) (top number)		Diastolic (mm Hg) (bottom number)
Optimal*	119 or lower	and	79 or lower
Normal	129 or lower	and	84 or lower
High-normal	130 to 139	or	85 to 89
Hypertension			
Stage 1†	140 to 159	or	90 to 99
Stage 2†	160 to 179	or	100 to 109
Stage 3†	180 or higher	or	110 or higher

*Optimal means the preferred range in terms of cardiovascular risk.
†Based on the average of two or more readings taken at each of two or more visits after an initial screening. Systolic hypertension is a major risk factor for cardiovascular disease, even without elevated diastolic pressure, especially in older people.
Source: National Institutes of Health, 1997. Numbers are expressed in millimeters of mercury.

controlled conditions permits more accurate observations of how you're doing over time.

If you have high blood pressure, your treatment plan might include measuring your blood pressure at home. See Chapter 10 for detailed instructions on home monitoring.

What's high blood pressure?

When the complex system that regulates your blood pressure doesn't work as it's supposed to, too much pressure can develop within your arteries. Increased pressure in your arteries that continues on a persistent basis is called high blood pressure.

The medical term for the condition is *hypertension,* meaning high tension in your arteries. Hypertension doesn't mean nervous tension, as many people believe. You can be a calm, relaxed person and still have high blood pressure.

Your blood pressure is considered high if your systolic pressure is consistently 140 mm Hg or higher, your diastolic pressure is consistently 90 mm Hg or higher, or both. Doctors traditionally assumed that diastolic blood pressure — the pressure between heartbeats — was a better indicator of health risks associated with elevated blood pressure than systolic pressure — the pressure when your heart contracts. But that's no longer believed to be the case. Studies have shown that a high systolic reading is a more important and more serious warning sign of potential health risks, especially in older adults. For people in this age group, controlling systolic pressure leads to important health benefits.

There are three separate stages of high blood pressure, based on increasing severity. They're referred to simply as stages 1, 2 and 3. The terms *mild* and *moderate* are no longer used to define levels of high blood pressure to avoid the possibility that people will mistakenly believe mild or moderate high blood pressure isn't serious.

High blood pressure generally develops slowly. In most instances, people start out with normal blood pressure that progresses to high-normal blood pressure and, eventually, to stage 1 high blood pressure. Most people with uncontrolled high blood pressure have stage 1 hypertension — very few have stage 3.

Left untreated, high blood pressure can damage many of your body's organs and tissues. The higher the blood pressure stage — and the longer it goes untreated — the greater the risk that injury will occur. However, even stage 1 high blood pressure can be harmful if it continues over a period of several months to years. When it's coupled with other factors known to be detrimental to your health, such as diabetes, obesity or tobacco use, your risk for injury from high blood pressure is even greater.

Incidentally, an old piece of conventional wisdom said that an ideal systolic blood pressure was 100 plus your age. That's not true. Following this adage as you age can deceive you into thinking that high blood pressure — even in stages 1, 2 and 3 — is normal.

Signs and symptoms

High blood pressure is called the silent killer because it often doesn't produce any signs or symptoms to warn you that you have a problem.

People sometimes take headaches, dizziness or nosebleeds as warning signs of increased blood pressure. A few people may experience more nosebleeds than usual or some dizziness when their blood pressure rises. But you shouldn't rely on a headache as a warning sign of high blood pressure. A study found no association between headaches and elevated blood pressure. Generally, most people don't experience any signs or symptoms.

You can have high blood pressure for years without ever knowing it. In fact, about 15 million Americans right now have no idea that their blood pressure is too high. The condition is most often discovered during a routine physical examination. Signs and symptoms typically don't occur until high blood pressure has advanced to a higher — possibly life-threatening — stage. However, even some people with stage 3 high blood pressure don't experience any signs or symptoms.

Other signs and symptoms sometimes associated with high blood pressure, such as excessive perspiration, muscle cramps, frequent urination or rapid or irregular heartbeats (palpitations), generally are caused by other conditions that can lead to high blood pressure.

When your blood pressure drops too low

Generally, the lower your blood pressure reading, the better. But in some cases, your blood pressure can drop too low, just as it can rise too high. Low blood pressure, called hypotension, can be life-threatening if it falls to dangerously low levels. However, this is rare.

Chronic low blood pressure — blood pressure that's below normal but not hazardously so — is fairly common. It can result from various factors, including high blood pressure medications, complications of diabetes and the second trimester of pregnancy.

A potentially dangerous side effect of chronic low blood pressure is postural hypotension, a condition in which you feel dizzy or faint when you stand too quickly. When you stand, the force of gravity causes blood to pool in your legs, which produces a sudden drop in blood pressure. Normally, the system that regulates your blood pressure counteracts the decrease almost simultaneously by narrowing your blood vessels and increasing the volume of blood flow from your heart.

If your blood pressure is chronically low, it takes longer for your body to respond to the change in pressure. Postural hypotension is more common with advanced age as nerve signals and regulatory system responses become slowed. The danger is that if you become too dizzy or lose consciousness, you can fall and injure yourself.

You can often avoid this problem by standing more slowly and holding on to something while you stand. Also, wait a few seconds after standing and before walking so that your body has time to adjust to the pressure change. Crossing your legs and squeezing your thighs together (like a scissors) while standing also may help by reducing blood flow to your legs.

Some older adults, particularly those on medication for high blood pressure, may be at risk of fainting or falling after eating a meal. The cause can be a drop in blood pressure. If you've experienced falling or fainting after a meal, take some preventive action. Eat slowly and avoid large meals. After you eat, rest for an hour.

See your doctor if you experience persistent dizziness or fainting. You may have another health condition that's causing the symptoms or that's making them worse than usual.

Complications

High blood pressure needs to be controlled because, over time, the excessive force on your artery walls can seriously damage many of your body's vital organs. Sites in your body typically most affected by high blood pressure include your arteries, heart, brain, kidneys and eyes.

Some of the complications listed below may require emergency treatment. For information on emergencies related to high blood pressure, see Chapter 12.

Your cardiovascular system

Complications from high blood pressure can affect the function of your arteries, your heart and other body systems (see illustration on page 14).

Arteriosclerosis. Healthy arteries are like healthy muscles. They're flexible, strong and elastic. Their inside lining is smooth so that blood can flow through them unrestricted. But over a period of years, too much pressure in your arteries can make the walls thick and stiff.

The term *arteriosclerosis* (ahr-tere-e-oh-skluh-RO-sis) means hardening of your arteries. It comes from the Greek word *sklerosis,* for "hardening." Sometimes, stiffened arteries in your forearms can actually be felt, and they may resemble small, hard pipes.

Atherosclerosis. High blood pressure can accelerate the accumulation of fatty deposits in and under the lining of artery walls. The name *atherosclerosis* (ath-ur-o-skluh-RO-sis) comes from the Greek word *ather* meaning "porridge," because the fatty deposits are soft and resemble porridge.

When the inner wall of an artery is damaged, blood cells called platelets often clump at the injury site. Fat deposits also gather at the site. Initially, the deposits are only streaks of fat-containing cells. As the deposits accumulate, they invade some of the deeper layers of your artery walls, causing the walls to become scarred. Large accumulations of fatty deposits are called plaques. Over time, plaques can harden.

The greatest danger from plaque formation is narrowing of the vessels. Organs and tissues that are served by these narrowed vessels don't get an adequate supply of blood. Your body responds to the

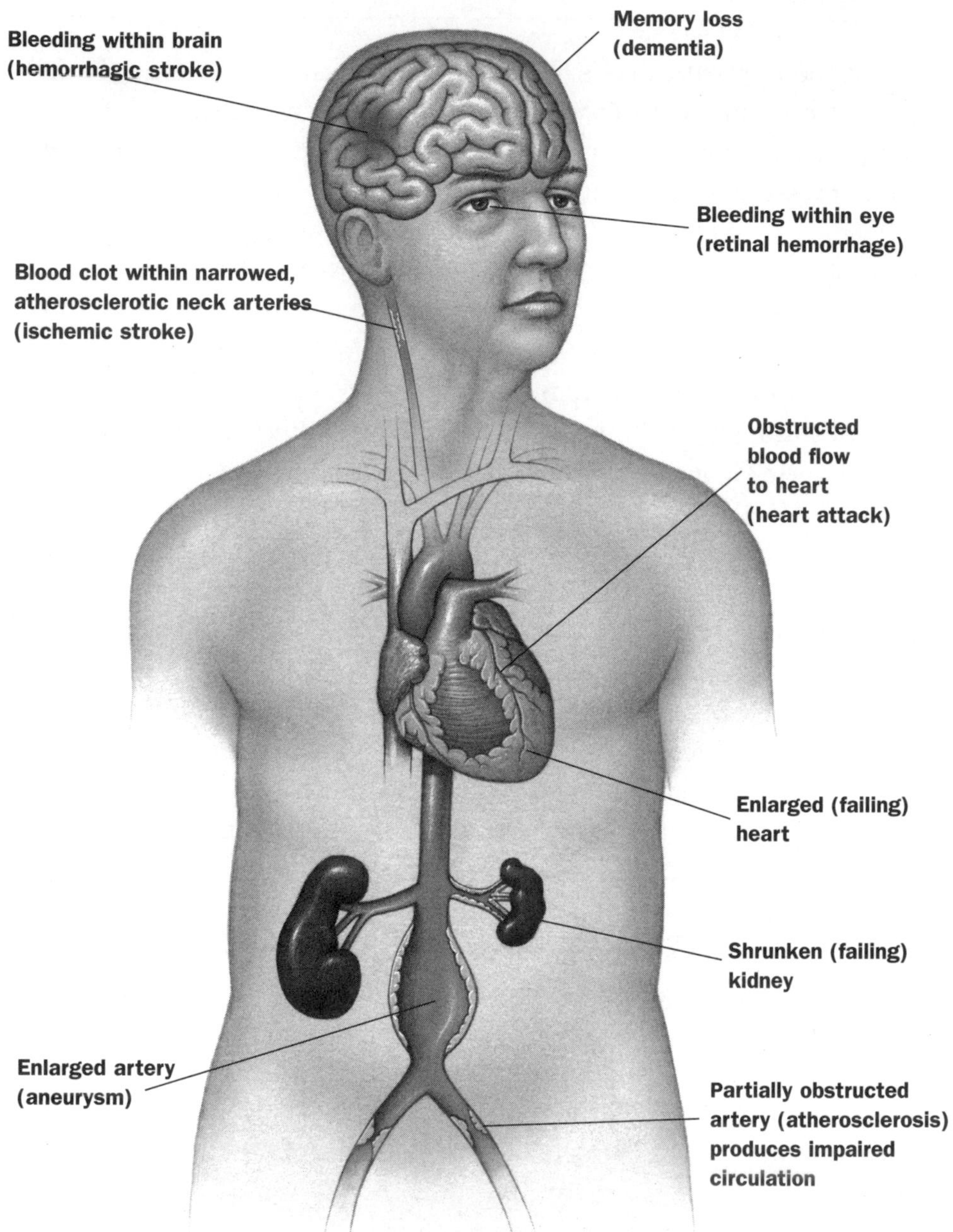

Left untreated, high blood pressure can damage tissues and organs throughout your body. Sites in your body most affected by high blood pressure include your arteries, heart, brain, kidneys and eyes.

shortage of blood by increasing blood pressure to maintain adequate blood flow. The increase in blood pressure leads to further blood vessel damage. Inflammation occurs around the plaques. Eventually plaques may break apart and block the artery, causing a blood clot, or travel with your blood until they lodge in a smaller artery.

Normal artery

Atherosclerotic plaques

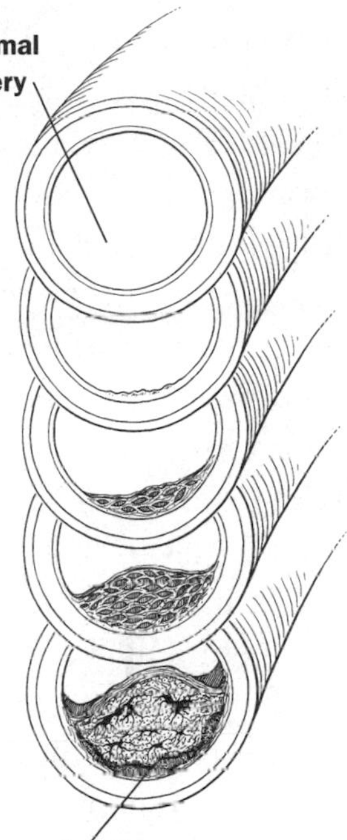

In atherosclerosis, deposits of plaque gradually accumulate in the lining of your arteries. As the deposits enlarge, blood circulation decreases and blood pressure increases. This increases your risk of heart attack, stroke and other vascular problems.

Arteriosclerosis and atherosclerosis can occur in arteries anywhere within your body. However, the diseases most often affect arteries in your heart, brain, kidneys, abdominal aorta and legs.

Aneurysm. When a blood vessel loses elasticity and weakens, a spot in its wall may bulge or balloon. This is called an aneurysm. Aneurysms most commonly occur in a brain artery or in the lower portion of the aorta that passes through your abdomen. The greatest danger with any aneurysm is that it may leak or burst, causing life-threatening bleeding.

In their early stages, aneurysms generally don't produce any symptoms. In more advanced stages, an aneurysm in a brain artery can lead to a severe headache that doesn't go away. An advanced abdominal aneurysm may cause constant pain in your abdomen or lower back. Occasionally, during a physical examination, a doctor can detect an abdominal aneurysm by feeling the pulsating vessel while pressing lightly on your abdomen. Sometimes, a clot lining the aneurysm wall breaks off and obstructs an artery downstream.

Coronary artery disease. The major cause of death in people with uncontrolled high blood pressure is one or more complications of coronary artery disease. Coronary artery disease refers to damage to the major arteries feeding your heart muscle. Accumulation of plaques in these arteries is common among people with high blood pressure.

Plaques reduce blood flow to your heart muscle, which can lead to a heart attack if your heart muscle is deprived of too much blood. This condition calls for an immediate trip to the emergency room for medication or angioplasty, a surgical procedure for repairing blood vessels. Lowering blood pressure has been shown to reduce the number of heart attacks by almost 30 percent.

Left ventricular hypertrophy. Blood pressure is like a weight or load that your heart muscle must lift. When your heart pumps blood into your aorta, it has to push the blood out against the pressure inside your arteries. The higher the pressure, the harder the muscle has to work. And your heart muscle, like any muscle, gets larger the harder it works.

Eventually, your heart can't keep up with the excessive workload and the muscular wall of its main pumping chamber (left ventricle) starts to thicken (hypertrophy). As the ventricle enlarges, it requires an increased supply of blood. But because high blood pressure also causes the blood vessels feeding your heart to narrow, the vessels often can't supply enough blood to meet your heart's needs. Control of high blood pressure can prevent — as well as reverse — this hypertrophy.

Heart failure. In this condition, your heart isn't able to pump the blood returning to it fast enough. As a result, fluid can back up and start to accumulate in your lungs, legs and other tissues, a condition called edema (uh-DEE-muh). Fluid in your lungs leads to shortness of breath. Buildup of fluid in your legs causes your feet and ankles to swell. With appropriate treatment of high blood pressure, the risk of heart failure can be reduced by 50 percent.

Your brain

High blood pressure significantly increases your odds of having a stroke. During more than 35 years of follow-up in the Framingham Heart Study, 56 percent of stroke in men and 66 percent in women were directly attributable to high blood pressure. The good news is that in people who received treatment for their high blood pressure, stroke risk dropped by 42 percent over 5 years.

A stroke, also called a brain attack, is a type of brain injury caused by a blocked or ruptured blood vessel in the brain that disturbs your brain's blood supply. There are two general types of stroke.

Ischemic strokes. Ischemic (is-KEM-ik) strokes are the most common, accounting for between 70 percent and 80 percent of all strokes. Ischemic strokes usually affect the portion of your brain called the cerebrum, which controls movement, language and senses.

These strokes result from a blood clot due to accumulation of plaques in an artery. The plaques roughen the inside of the blood vessel surface, forcing blood to flow around the plaques, which can trigger development of a blood clot. More than half of ischemic strokes are caused by stationary (thrombotic) blood clots that develop in the arteries leading from your heart to your brain.

A less common form of ischemic stroke occurs when a tiny piece of clotted blood breaks loose from an artery wall and is swept through larger arteries into smaller vessels in your brain. A clot that may have developed in a chamber in your heart can also break loose. If the moving (embolic) clot lodges in a small artery and blocks blood flow to a portion of your brain, a stroke occurs.

Sometimes the blood supply to the brain is disrupted only briefly — less than 24 hours. This is a transient ischemic attack (TIA), sometimes called a little stroke. A TIA is one warning sign of a possible impending stroke.

Hemorrhagic strokes. A hemorrhagic (hem-uh-RAJ-ik) stroke occurs when a blood vessel in the brain leaks or ruptures. Blood from the hemorrhage spills into surrounding brain tissue, damaging the tissue. Brain cells beyond the leak or rupture also are damaged because they're deprived of blood. One cause of a hemorrhagic stroke is an aneurysm. A small tear in a brain artery also can cause blood to leak.

Improved detection and treatment of high blood pressure throughout the past 40 years have contributed to a dramatic reduction in the number of strokes. When your blood pressure is lowered through appropriate treatment, your risk of stroke decreases remarkably — about 40 percent over a period of 2 to 5 years.

Even if you've had a stroke or TIA, lowering your blood pressure can prevent these problems from happening again.

In addition, clot-busting medications given within the first few hours after signs and symptoms of an ischemic stroke begin can greatly reduce disability from the stroke.

Dementia. Studies suggest that high blood pressure can lead to dementia, loss of memory and other mental ability. The risk of such dementia increases dramatically in people age 70 and older. After a diagnosis of high blood pressure, dementia can appear from a few years to several decades later. Recent evidence suggests that drug treatment to control high blood pressure may lower dementia risk.

Are you taking a daily aspirin?

High blood pressure increases your risk of other heart and blood vessel (cardiovascular) disease, such as heart attack and stroke. You can counteract this increased risk by taking a daily aspirin.

A primary cause of heart attack and stroke is accumulation of hard deposits (plaques) in your arteries. The deposits reduce the flow of blood and can cause blood to clot. Inflammation also may occur in arteries containing plaque deposits. Aspirin, a blood thinner, reduces the tendency of blood to clot and may reduce accompanying inflammation. The daily recommended dose is anywhere from 81 milligrams (mg), the amount found in a baby aspirin, to 325 mg, the amount found in an adult tablet.

Your blood pressure should be controlled before you start aspirin, so talk with your doctor first. To help prevent stomach irritation or bleeding that can occur from regular aspirin use, take aspirin with food and take enteric-coated aspirin tablets, which dissolve in your small intestine instead of your stomach.

Aspirin and other over-the-counter pain relievers can interact with prescription drugs in harmful ways. For important information about preventing drug interactions, see Chapter 11.

Your kidneys

About one-fifth of the blood pumped by your heart goes to your kidneys. Tiny filtering structures in your kidneys called nephrons filter out waste products in your blood, which are later excreted in the urine. Your kidneys control the balance of minerals, acids and water in your blood. In addition, they produce chemicals that control blood vessel size and function. High blood pressure can interfere with this intricate process.

When blood vessels in your kidneys develop atherosclerosis due to high blood pressure, blood flow to the nephrons is reduced and your kidneys can't eliminate all of the waste products in your blood. Over time, waste can build up in your blood and your kidneys can shrink and stop functioning. High blood pressure and diabetes are the most common causes of kidney failure.

When your kidneys stop functioning, you need to undergo kidney dialysis, and you may need a kidney transplant. Kidney dialysis is a process by which waste products in your blood are filtered out by machine.

Because part of the role of your kidneys is to help control blood pressure by regulating the amount of sodium and water in your blood, damage to your kidneys can worsen your high blood pressure. This can produce a destructive cycle that ultimately results in increasing blood pressure and a gradual failure of your kidneys to remove impurities from your blood.

Reducing blood pressure can slow the progression of kidney disease and reduce the likelihood of dialysis and transplant.

Your eyes

High blood pressure speeds the normal aging of tiny blood vessels in your eyes. In severe cases, it may even lead to vision loss.

Occasionally, a simple eye examination will lead to the discovery of high blood pressure. Shining a light into your eye makes tiny blood vessels in the back of your eye (retina) visible. In the early stages of high blood pressure, these tiny arteries can thicken and narrow. Eventually, the vessels can develop blockages that compress nearby veins, interfering with blood flow in the veins.

High blood pressure can also cause tiny blood vessels in your retina to tear and leak blood and fluid into surrounding tissue. In severe cases, the nerve that carries visual signals from your retina to your brain (optic nerve) may start to swell. This can result in loss of vision. This damage to the retina is largely preventable with control of high blood pressure.

Wrap-up

Key points to remember:

- Blood pressure is necessary for smooth flow of blood through your heart and blood vessels.
- Both numbers in a blood pressure reading are important.
- High blood pressure refers to systolic blood pressure that's consistently 140 millimeters of mercury (mm Hg) or higher, diastolic pressure that's consistently 90 mm Hg or higher, or both.
- An estimated 50 million Americans have high blood pressure, but only about a quarter have their disease under control.
- High blood pressure is often called the silent killer because it typically doesn't produce any symptoms.
- Left untreated, high blood pressure can lead to stroke, heart attack, heart and kidney failure, blindness and dementia.
- By controlling high blood pressure, you significantly reduce your risk of disability or death related to the disease.

Chapter 2

Are you at risk?

With any disease, you naturally want to know what causes it. Why does it occur in some people but not in others? Unfortunately, for most people with high blood pressure, the reason for the condition is unknown.

However, it's clear that certain factors can put you at greater risk for high blood pressure. By knowing what these factors are, you can take steps to minimize your risk and possibly prevent the disease from occurring.

Essential high blood pressure

There are two forms of high blood pressure — essential and secondary. Essential is the most common. Between 90 percent and 95 percent of people with high blood pressure have the essential form, also known as primary high blood pressure.

Essential high blood pressure differs from secondary high blood pressure in that it has no obvious cause. Among the large majority of people who have high blood pressure, it's difficult to pinpoint exactly what's triggering the increase in their blood pressure. Researchers are studying the possibility that genes play a role in the development of the condition. And while there are rare instances in which single-gene disorders affect sodium metabolism and cause high blood pressure, research indicates that most high blood pressure is a complex illness that doesn't follow the classic rules of inheritance. Instead of stemming from a single defective gene, it appears to be a multifaceted disorder that involves interaction between several genes. In addition, factors including weight, sodium use and physical activity also appear to interact with genetic factors. Because of this, it's doubtful that researchers will be able to link a specific genetic defect to all essential hypertension.

More likely, essential high blood pressure results from a combination of factors related to:

- Motion (widening and narrowing) of your blood vessels
- Increased fluid in your blood
- Functioning of your blood flow sensors (baroreceptors)
- Production of chemicals that influence how your blood vessels function
- Secretion of hormones
- Volume of blood pumped by your heart
- Nerve control of your cardiovascular system

Risk factors

Certain genetic traits and lifestyle habits play an important role in the development of essential high blood pressure. Generally, the more of these risk factors you have, the greater the odds that you'll have high blood pressure during your lifetime. Most risk factors you can control, others you can't.

Things you can't change

There are four major unmodifiable risk factors for high blood pressure that you can't control.

Race. High blood pressure occurs far more frequently in blacks of African-American descent than in any other racial group in the United States. Data from the Third National Health and Nutrition Examination Survey (NHANES III, 1988-1991) showed that 40 percent more blacks than whites had high blood pressure. Among Americans age 18 and older, 32.4 percent of blacks versus 23.3 percent of whites had high blood pressure. The highest rates of high blood pressure in the United States were among blacks living in the southeastern states. High blood pressure in blacks generally develops at an earlier age than in whites. Plus, it's usually more pronounced and tends to progress more rapidly. For these reasons, blacks have the highest death rate from complications related to the condition. According to the American Heart Association, 30 percent of all deaths in black men and 20 percent of deaths in black women with hypertension may be attributable to high blood pressure.

Age. Your risk of high blood pressure increases with age. Although high blood pressure can occur at any age, it's most often detected in people age 35 or older. Among black and white Americans age 65 or older, more than half have high blood pressure.

It's fairly common for your blood pressure to increase slightly with age. This is often due to natural changes affecting your heart, blood vessels and hormones. However, when these changes are coupled with other risk factors, they can lead to the development of high blood pressure.

Family history. High blood pressure tends to run in families. If one of your parents has high blood pressure, you have about a 25 percent chance of developing it during your lifetime. If both your mother and father have high blood pressure, you have about a 60 percent chance of acquiring the disease. Studies of twins and of people within the same family who have high blood pressure show that an inherited component may play a role in some cases of the disease.

However, just because high blood pressure exists in your family doesn't mean you're destined to get it. Even in families in which high blood pressure is prevalent, some blood relatives never develop the disease.

Sex. Among young and middle-age adults, men are more likely to have high blood pressure than are women. Later on, the reverse is true. After age 55, when most women are beyond menopause, high blood pressure becomes more common in women than in men.

Among Americans age 18 and older, 34 percent of black men and 31 percent of black women have high blood pressure. That compares with 25 percent of white men and 21 percent of white women who have hypertension. For Hispanics, the figures are about 23 percent for men and about 22 percent for women.

Among Asian-Americans and Pacific Islanders, the prevalence is about 10 percent of men and 8 percent of women. Among American Indians, about 27 percent of men and 27 percent of women have high blood pressure.

Things you can change

These are modifiable risk factors for high blood pressure that you can control.

Obesity. Being overweight increases your risk of development of high blood pressure for several reasons. The more body mass you have, the more blood you need to supply oxygen and nutrients to your tissues. That means the volume of blood being circulated through your blood vessels is increased, creating extra force on your artery walls.

Excess weight can also increase your heart rate and the level of insulin in your blood. Increased insulin causes your body to retain sodium and water.

In addition, some people who are overweight follow a diet that's too high in fat, especially saturated and trans fats. These fats promote the accumulation of fatty deposits (plaques) in your arteries, causing narrowing of your arteries. For most people, a diet contains too much fat if more than 30 percent of total daily calories come from fat.

Insulin resistance syndrome, or metabolic syndrome. Your digestive system normally breaks down some of the food you eat into sugar (glucose). Your blood then carries the glucose to all of the cells of your body, where it's used for energy. Insulin, a hormone produced in your pancreas, is needed to allow glucose to enter your cells. In some people, however, there's a diminished ability to respond to insulin. This is called insulin resistance syndrome, or metabolic syndrome, formerly known as syndrome X. With this condition, your body makes more and more insulin in an effort to help glucose get into your cells.

This extra insulin helps maintain normal blood glucose levels for a while. But eventually your pancreas is unable to overcome insulin resistance. Glucose accumulates in your body, leading to type 2 diabetes (formerly called adult-onset or noninsulin-dependent diabetes.)

Even before you develop diabetes, years of excess insulin in your system can lead to other health problems. Key signs of insulin resistance syndrome include obesity, high blood pressure, high triglycerides (a type of blood fat) and low levels of high-density lipoprotein (HDL) cholesterol (the "good" cholesterol).

Doctors believe the risk of insulin resistance is partly inherited. However, being overweight and inactive also are major contributors. A study published in 2002 that included more than 8,800 adults age 20 and older found that nearly 22 percent had insulin resistance syndrome. The highest prevalence — nearly 32 percent — was in Hispanics.

Strategies for managing insulin resistance syndrome include exercising, losing weight, eating a fiber-rich diet and stopping smoking. If these aren't enough to curb insulin resistance, your doctor may prescribe medication.

Inactivity. Lack of physical activity increases your risk of high blood pressure by increasing your risk of becoming overweight. People who are inactive also tend to have higher heart rates, and their heart muscle has to work harder with each contraction. The harder and more often your heart has to pump, the greater is the force being exerted on your arteries.

Tobacco use. The chemicals in tobacco can damage the lining of your artery walls, making them more prone to the accumulation of plaques.

Nicotine in tobacco also makes your heart work harder by temporarily constricting your blood vessels and increasing your heart rate and blood pressure. These effects occur because of increased hormone production during tobacco use, including increased levels of the hormone epinephrine (adrenaline).

In addition, carbon monoxide in cigarette smoke replaces oxygen in your blood. This can increase blood pressure by forcing your heart to work harder to supply adequate oxygen to your body's organs and tissues. For details on stopping smoking, see Chapter 8.

Sodium sensitivity. Your body needs a certain amount of the mineral sodium to maintain proper cell chemistry. A common source of sodium is table salt (sodium chloride), which is composed of about 40 percent sodium and 60 percent chloride.

However, some people are more sensitive to the presence of sodium in their blood than are others. People who are sodium sensitive retain sodium more easily, leading to fluid retention and increased blood pressure. If you're in this group, excessive sodium in your diet can increase your chances for having high blood pressure. Remember that most dietary salt comes as an added ingredient in foods, so read labels carefully. For more on salt, see Chapter 5.

It's estimated that up to 60 percent of Americans with high blood pressure are sodium sensitive. Among blacks, the percentage is higher. Only about 15 percent to 25 percent of people without high blood pressure have sodium sensitivity. As you age, your sensitivity to sodium often becomes more pronounced.

Unfortunately, this sensitivity is difficult to assess. And since there's no health reason to consume excess salt, almost all of us can benefit from reducing sodium intake.

Low potassium. Potassium is a mineral that helps balance the amount of sodium in cell fluids. It gets rid of excess sodium in your cells by way of your kidneys, which filter out the sodium to be excreted in your urine. If your diet doesn't include enough potassium or your body isn't able to retain a proper amount, too much sodium can accumulate, increasing your risk of developing high blood pressure.

Low potassium levels also stimulate release of aldosterone, a hormone that increases retention of sodium and water, raising the risk of high blood pressure. For more on eating well, see Chapter 6.

Excessive alcohol. It's estimated that excessive alcohol consumption contributes to between 5 percent and 20 percent of all cases of high blood pressure. Consuming three or more drinks of alcohol per day approximately doubles your risk of developing high blood pressure. Exactly how or why alcohol increases blood pressure isn't fully understood. But it's known that over time, heavy drinking can damage your heart and other organs.

The safest course is to drink moderately or not at all. For most men, moderate drinking means no more than 2 alcoholic drinks a day. For women, the limit is 1 drink daily.

The fattening of America

America's waistline continues to expand at an alarming rate. It's now estimated that 120 million adults are either overweight or obese. That's up from 97 million in the 1990s and represents nearly two-thirds of the adult population. Overweight is defined as having a body mass index (BMI) between 25.0 and 29.9. Obesity is defined as having a BMI of 30 or greater.

According to reports published in the October 9, 2002, issue of the *Journal of the American Medical Association*, comparing the periods 1988 to 1994 and 1999 to 2000, the rates of overweight and obesity increased for both genders and across all races and ethnic and age groups. The reports indicated that 64.5 percent of adults are overweight and 30.5 percent are obese. Those figures are up from the previous period when 55.9 percent of adults were overweight and 22.9 percent were obese.

Adults aren't the only ones putting on excess weight. The prevalence of overweight among 12- to 19-year-olds went from 10.5 percent to 15.5 percent. The prevalence went from 11.3 percent to 15.3 percent for children ages 6 to 11 years, and from 7.2 percent to 10.4 percent for ages 2 to 5 years. The prevalence of overweight in children is especially high among Hispanic and black adolescents.

Overweight and obesity increase with age. The latest figures show that nearly 40 percent of women and nearly 36 percent of men between ages 60 and 74 are obese.

Excess weight is second only to smoking as a leading cause of preventable death in the United States. About 300,000 U.S. deaths a year are associated with overweight or obesity. In comparison, 430,000 deaths a year are associated with cigarette smoking.

Only 3 percent of all Americans meet at least four of the five federal dietary recommendations for consumption of grains, fruits, vegetables, dairy products and meats.

Only 22 percent of Americans meet the recommendations to engage in at least 30 minutes of moderate physical activity at least five times a week. Forty percent of adults engage in no leisure-time physical activity at all.

Note that these are only general recommendations for moderate drinking. Guidelines for individuals may vary. For example, small-frame men and people age 65 and older should limit themselves to 1 drink daily. For more on alcohol and high blood pressure, see Chapter 8.

Stress. Stress doesn't cause persistent high blood pressure. But high levels of stress can lead to a temporary, dramatic increase. If temporary stress episodes occur often enough, they can damage your blood vessels, heart and kidneys in the same manner as persistent high blood pressure.

Stress can also promote high blood pressure by causing you to develop unhealthy habits known to increase the risk of hypertension. Some people bothered by stress turn to smoking, alcohol or overeating to relieve their stress.

Other illnesses

You may also be at increased risk of developing high blood pressure if you have a chronic illness. Illnesses that can contribute to increased blood pressure or make high blood pressure more difficult to control are described here.

In addition, women, children, older adults and people in certain ethnic groups may have unique concerns in controlling blood pressure. For details, see chapter 12.

High cholesterol. High levels of cholesterol, a fat-like substance in your blood, promote the development of plaques in your arteries (atherosclerosis), causing them to narrow and be less able to dilate. These changes can increase your blood pressure.

Diabetes. Too much sugar in your blood can damage many of your organs and tissues, leading to atherosclerosis, kidney disease and coronary artery disease. These diseases all affect your blood pressure.

Sleep apnea. Obstructive sleep apnea is a severe form of snoring that interrupts breathing during sleep. Several studies have established a link between the interrupted breathing and temporary reduction in oxygen supply that accompanies sleep apnea and the onset of high blood pressure. It's thought that long-term nervous system and cell responses to sleep apnea may cause blood vessel problems that eventually lead to high blood pressure.

It's not always evident when you have sleep apnea. But if you consistently have difficulty getting a restful night's sleep and have trouble staying awake during the day, talk with your doctor. Overweight and obesity contribute to the risk of sleep apnea.

Treatment may include using supplemental oxygen while you sleep. It's been shown to provide small decreases in blood pressure in people with sleep apnea.

Heart failure. If your heart muscle is damaged or weakened, possibly due to a heart attack, it has to work harder to pump blood. High blood pressure that's uncontrolled increases demand on your weakened heart and complicates the treatment of both conditions.

Other indicators for increased cardiovascular risk include changes in blood circulation in your retina, a thickening of the wall of your heart's left ventricle (left ventricular hypertrophy), changes in the level of creatinine (a chemical excreted by the kidneys) in your blood and the amount of protein in your urine. Treatment of high blood pressure can reverse or retard the progression of these risk factors.

A multiplying effect

Risk factors usually don't function independently. They often interact with each other in important ways. For example, if you have two risk factors — you're overweight and you're inactive — your odds of having high blood pressure are much higher than if you have either one alone.

By the same token, working to reduce one risk factor may have benefits for others. Your total reduction in risk may be more than the sum of that one factor alone.

Remember: The word *risk* refers to odds or chances — not to inevitability or guarantees. Clearly, risk factors affect your chances for having high blood pressure. But having one or more risk factors doesn't guarantee that you'll get high blood pressure. By the same token, you could develop high blood pressure even if you have no risk factors. The bottom line is that by reducing the modifiable risks, you lower your chance of getting high blood pressure and its complications.

Secondary high blood pressure

In about 5 percent to 10 percent of high blood pressure cases, a cause can be identified. This is called secondary high blood pressure because the condition is due to — or is secondary to — another disease or disorder. This condition is also called secondary hypertension.

Secondary high blood pressure usually has a more rapid onset and causes higher blood pressure than essential, or primary, high blood pressure, which generally develops gradually over many years.

Unlike essential high blood pressure, secondary high blood pressure can sometimes be cured. When the underlying disease or condition is corrected, blood pressure typically decreases. In some people, blood pressure may return to normal.

Major causes

Secondary hypertension can be caused by a number of different conditions. Here are some of the main causes.

Kidney problems. Kidneys are important in the regulation of blood pressure, and kidney problems account for a large share of secondary hypertension.

Polycystic kidneys, an inherited disorder, and other kidney diseases such as diabetic kidney disease, nephritis and scleroderma, result in kidney damage that eventually can lead to chronic renal failure. Your kidneys no longer get rid of salt, water and waste products normally, and the scarring and narrowing of blood vessels contribute to raising your blood pressure. Damaged kidneys also may release hormones and other chemicals that raise your blood pressure.

If kidney disease is suspected, your doctor may take a careful family history to see if other family members have had kidney problems, as they often run in families. Your doctor will also do a thorough physical examination, including examining your abdomen, because large cysts in your kidneys sometimes can be felt through the abdominal wall. Urine and blood tests may indicate kidney malfunction, and ultrasound examinations, computerized tomography (CT) scans or magnetic resonance imaging (MRI) examinations of your kidneys can reveal cysts or scars caused by disease.

In some instances, surgery may be necessary to reduce the size and number of cysts in order to decrease pressure from the cysts on the remaining normal kidney tissue. In severe cases, kidney transplantation may be needed.

Obstruction of the renal artery. Obstruction of a renal artery, the main vessel supplying blood to each kidney, also can cause secondary hypertension. The obstruction is most often due to narrowing of the artery caused by atherosclerosis. When severe, the kidney downstream of the narrowing may shrink and scar irreversibly.

Narrowed kidney arteries can also be caused by a condition called fibromuscular dysplasia. In this condition the middle layer of the kidney artery wall (media) is thickened, narrowing the artery. The artery may have narrowed sections alternating with dilated or widened sections, which may become small aneurysms. One or both kidneys may be affected.

Arterial narrowing can also impair kidney function and lead to production of a hormone that raises the blood pressure in your body. The high blood pressure in such cases often responds to drug treatment. If it doesn't respond, however, or if kidney function is severely impaired, the obstructions may be opened with catheters and stents similar to those used in treating narrowed coronary arteries. Surgery may also be used to bypass the obstructed vessels.

Sometimes, narrowed kidney arteries can be diagnosed with a stethoscope — turbulent blood flow through the narrowed artery produces a distinctive sound, called a bruit (BRU-we). Narrowed arteries and changes in your kidneys are also detected through examinations, including ultrasound, CT, MRI and nuclear scanning. In nuclear scanning, a radioactive material called an isotope is injected into a vein. Images taken as the isotope circulates through your renal artery can reveal altered blood flow and function of the affected kidney.

Coarctation of the aorta. This is a narrowing of the primary blood vessel supplying blood from your heart to your body. Coarctation usually occurs in the portion of the aorta in your chest and rarely in your abdomen. It's usually detected at birth and repaired in the first 1 to 3 years of life. Occasionally, a person reaches adulthood before the condition is detected.

The narrowed aorta results in high blood pressure in your arms and low blood pressure in your legs. This can be determined by feeling the artery in your groin and at your wrist simultaneously and noting a delay in the arrival of the pulse at your groin. The pulse in your groin also feels less forceful than normal. A chest X-ray and images of the aorta made with ultrasound or MRI can establish the diagnosis.

In most cases, the coarctation is repaired surgically. The narrowed portion of the aorta is removed, and the ends of the aorta are sewn back together. In cases in which the narrowing recurs after the surgical repair, the narrow area can be stretched open using a balloon on the end of a catheter (balloon dilatation). The catheter is inserted through the artery in your groin during a cardiac catheterization procedure. If the balloon dilatation fails to permanently expand the narrow area of the aorta, a metallic stent may be inserted through a catheter to hold the narrow area open. These stents are approved for use in such cases, and while their long-term success is unknown, the results so far are good.

Pheochromocytoma. This is a tumor of the inner layer (medulla) of the adrenal gland. You have two adrenal glands, one atop each of your kidneys. These tumors, which can also occur in other parts of your body and may be in multiple locations, secrete the hormones epinephrine and norepinephrine as well as other chemicals.

Pheochromocytoma almost always causes prominent signs and symptoms. If you have one of these types of tumors, you may experience spells of sudden severe headache, heart palpitations and profuse perspiration, during which time you appear pale. These spells may last minutes to an hour and recur daily or very infrequently. Your blood pressure is almost always markedly elevated during the spell, and may also be elevated between spells.

Diagnostic tests include blood and urine tests and imaging of the tumor by CT, MRI or isotopes. Genetic tests also may be helpful, because this condition can run in families. The tumor is rarely malignant and can be removed by surgery.

Thyroid dysfunction.

Hyperthyroidism. Overproduction of thyroid hormone is called hyperthyroidism and may elevate your systolic blood pressure and heart rate. Signs and symptoms include:

- Nervousness
- Excessive perspiration
- Heat intolerance
- Palpitations
- Tremor
- Fatigue
- Weight loss
- Prominent eyes (exophthalmos)
- Enlarged thyroid or presence of nodules on your thyroid

Hyperthyroidism may run in families. The condition is diagnosed through blood tests and tests using radioactive isotopes. Treatment, which restores blood pressure to normal, includes medication, radioactive iodine and, in rare circumstances, surgery.

Hypothyroidism. Underproduction of thyroid hormone, or hypothyroidism, also can cause high blood pressure — both systolic and diastolic. Signs and symptoms include:

- Cold intolerance
- Fatigue
- Slowing of body functions
- Weight gain
- Coarse skin
- Low, husky voice
- Puffiness about your eyes, legs and hands

This condition may occur after treatment of an overactive thyroid or inflammation of the thyroid gland. It's diagnosed by taking a history, performing a physical examination and conducting blood tests. Treatment with thyroid hormone (thyroxin) usually restores your body to normal.

Cushing's syndrome and aldosteronism. These disorders are due to hormones produced by the outer layer (cortex) of the adrenal gland.

Cushing's syndrome is the result of excessive amounts of cortisol. The cortisol can either come from medication, such as prednisone, or be produced by your adrenal gland. The excess cortisol can also be caused by increased production of another hormone by your pituitary gland, or various other tumors that stimulate its release. Adrenal gland disorders can run in families.

Excess cortisol can cause numerous changes, including:

- Increased fatty deposits on your face (moon face), neck and trunk
- Thinned skin, purple stretch marks, easy bruising and excessive hair growth
- Emotional instability
- Weight gain
- High blood pressure
- Weakness
- Diabetes
- Osteoporosis

Diagnostic tests include blood and urine tests, specialized endocrine testing, CT scans or MRI examinations. If pituitary disease is suspected, a special blood sampling test may be needed. Treatment is directed at reducing the excess cortisol and can include eliminating or changing medications and surgery if the problem is internal in origin.

Excessive secretion of aldosterone from your adrenal gland (aldosteronism), sometimes caused by a tumor in the adrenal cortex, also can cause high blood pressure. Aldosterone causes you to retain sodium and water and also results in loss of potassium by your kidneys. However, you won't experience generalized swelling. It also can contribute to thickening of your heart. Your blood pressure can be very high at times.

If you have aldosteronism, which can run in families, you may have high blood pressure that is resistant to ordinary drug treatment. A low potassium level in your blood is a clue. Other diagnostic steps include urine, endocrine and genetic tests, and CT scans or MRI examinations. Treatment includes drugs to block the action of aldosterone and surgery to remove the tumor in your adrenal gland.

Preeclampsia. Blood pressure is measured and a urinalysis is routinely done during pregnancy, particularly after midpregnancy. Sometime after the twentieth week, about 6 percent to 8 percent of pregnant women develop a condition called preeclampsia (pre-e-KLAMP-se-uh). It's characterized by a significant increase in blood pressure and excess protein in the urine. Left untreated, it can lead to serious, even deadly complications for the baby and its mother.

After the baby is born, blood pressure usually returns to normal within several days to several weeks. Preeclampsia may indicate the possibility of future nonpregnancy hypertension for the mother or a repeat of the problem during a subsequent pregnancy. Preeclampsia is discussed further on page 176.

Illicit drug use. Street drugs, such as cocaine and amphetamines, can lead to high blood pressure by narrowing the arteries that supply blood to your heart, increasing your heart rate or damaging your heart muscle.

Medications. A number of drugs can increase blood pressure in some people. Over-the-counter medications (OTC) that may have this effect include:

- Cold remedies
- Nasal decongestants (including sprays)
- Appetite suppressants
- Nonsteroidal anti-inflammatory drugs (NSAIDs)

Prescription medications also can affect blood pressure, including:

- Steroids (Deltasone, Medrol)
- Tricyclic antidepressants (Asendin, Elavil, others)
- Cyclosporine (Neoral, Sandimmune, others)
- Epoetin alpha (Epogen, Procrit)
- COX-2 inhibitors (Celebrex, Vioxx, Bextra)

Birth control pills may also increase blood pressure slightly. In a few cases, though, the increase may be more dramatic, triggering the development of high blood pressure. Drospirenone, a component of a newer contraceptive pill (Yasmin), can cause the body to retain potassium and interfere with certain medications for high blood pressure.

Sibutramine (Meridia), a prescription drug used to manage obesity, substantially increases blood pressure in some people.

Herbal supplements. These products can contain ingredients that may not mix safely with prescription or nonprescription drugs. Also, some medical conditions increase the risks of taking supplements.

One supplement of great concern is ephedra, also known by its traditional Chinese medicine name, ma-huang. Herbal products containing ephedra are marketed in the United States to promote weight loss, increase energy and enhance athletic performance. However, ephedra contains ephedrine, a chemical stimulant that has been linked to high blood pressure, as well as a number of other serious health problems.

It's very important to tell your doctor about all medication you're currently taking — prescription drugs, nonprescription drugs and herbal products. This is especially important if you're taking medication for high blood pressure. For more information on safe use of medications, see Chapter 11.

Identifying secondary high blood pressure

With primary high blood pressure, no obvious cause can be found and symptoms often aren't present. You may not know you have high blood pressure until your doctor checks it. In secondary high blood pressure, the symptoms of the underlying condition may be what brought you to the doctor.

If you discover you have high blood pressure, your doctor may inquire about your family history and past medical history. He or she likely will look for evidence of heart attack, heart disease, hardening of the arteries, weight changes, leg pain with exercise, weakness and fatigue. Your doctor may also check for signs or symptoms of conditions such as pheochromocytoma or thyroid dysfunction, which can cause secondary hypertension. For more details on what your doctor may look for during the exam, see "Physical examination" on page 47.

Prevention

High blood pressure is often preventable. And efforts continue to be made within the medical community to prevent the disease, as well as to treat it. These efforts are aimed mainly at people with high-normal blood pressure.

For years, as long as your blood pressure was below the cutoff for being high, it was considered acceptable. That's no longer true. Doctors now know that high-normal blood pressure often leads to high blood pressure. And they've found that even high-normal blood pressure may increase your risk of cardiovascular disease.

High-normal blood pressure refers to persistent systolic readings between 130 and 139 millimeters of mercury (mm Hg), diastolic readings between 85 and 89 mm Hg, or both. If your blood pressure is within these ranges, take steps to lower it until it reaches a normal or, ideally, optimal level. (See "Classification of blood pressure" on page 9.)

You can reduce your blood pressure and your risk of other cardiovascular diseases by eliminating or changing risk factors that you can control. They include:

- Losing weight, if you're overweight
- Becoming more physically active
- Eating a healthy diet
- Stopping tobacco use
- Limiting alcohol

People with diabetes, heart or kidney disease should aim for a blood pressure of less than 130/80 mm Hg. In addition to lifestyle changes to lower blood pressure, these people often require medications.

Why act now?

You may wonder why it's so important to prevent high blood pressure. Why not simply wait for it to develop and then treat it? There are many reasons why it's better to act early instead of later.

Generally, the younger you are when you change your lifestyle, the better your chances of succeeding. The longer you're involved in an unhealthy habit, the more difficult it is to change it.

Even if you control your high blood pressure after the condition develops, you still have a higher risk of a heart attack or stroke than people who have never had high blood pressure. Even with successful treatment of blood pressure, changes in the heart and arteries that took place before your diagnosis may not reverse completely to normal.

Wrap-up

Key points to remember:

- There are two forms of high blood pressure — essential (primary) and secondary. The cause of essential high blood pressure, the most common type, isn't known. Secondary high blood pressure results from an underlying illness or condition. This form of high blood pressure is often curable.
- Certain genetic traits or lifestyle factors place you at increased risk for the development of high blood pressure. Generally, the more of them you have, the greater your risk.
- You may be able to prevent high blood pressure by eliminating or reducing risk factors that you can change.
- If you have high-normal blood pressure, reducing it to a normal or optimal level can keep you from developing high blood pressure and cardiovascular diseases.

Chapter 3

Diagnosis and treatment

Unlike many other health conditions, high blood pressure rarely produces any signs or symptoms to warn you that something's wrong. Most people who have uncontrolled high blood pressure feel and look just fine.

That's why it's important to have your blood pressure checked at least every 2 years. Otherwise, you could be living with increased blood pressure for years and never know it.

It's during a routine medical examination that most people first learn their blood pressure is too high. Fortunately, diagnosing high blood pressure is a relatively simple and straightforward process. It involves having your blood pressure measured periodically over a few weeks or months to see if it remains increased.

As part of the diagnostic process, your doctor likely will ask you questions about your health and your family's health, do a physical examination and have you undergo some routine tests. These steps are done to determine whether your organs have been damaged and to prevent additional health problems associated with high blood pressure. Results from the history, examination and tests are also important in deciding how best to treat your condition. (See "Getting an evaluation" on page 44.)

The two methods for reducing and controlling high blood pressure are lifestyle changes and medication. Whether you'll need medication depends on your blood pressure stage, your risk of other health problems and whether the disease has caused any organ damage.

Measuring your blood pressure

Determining your blood pressure levels is a fairly easy procedure. Here's how a measurement is taken.

A sphygmomanometer (sfig-mo-muh-NOM-uh-tur) is the device that measures blood pressure. It includes an inflatable arm cuff with an attached air pump and a column of mercury or a standardized pressure gauge.

During a blood pressure measurement, the cuff is wrapped around your upper arm. Air is then pumped into the cuff by squeezing the bulb on the air pump. The cuff is inflated until the pressure inside it reaches a level well above your systolic pressure (upper number). This causes the main artery in your arm (brachial artery) to collapse, cutting off blood flow to the rest of your arm. When the artery collapses, no sounds are heard through a stethoscope that's placed over the artery, just below the cuff.

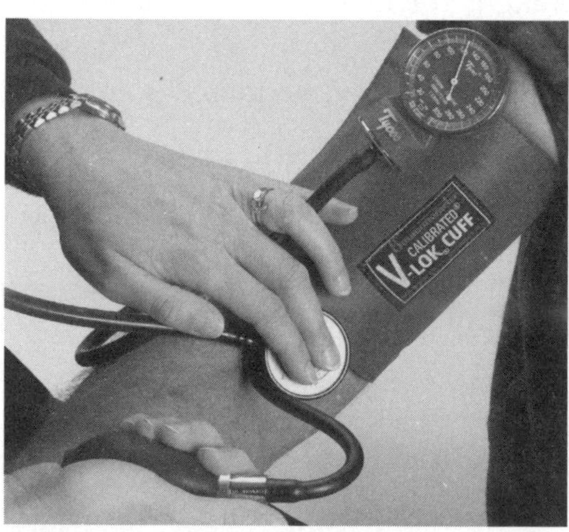

During a blood pressure reading, a doctor or nurse listens for two sounds indicating your systolic and diastolic pressures.

Air is then slowly released from the cuff, gradually reducing pressure on the artery. As soon as pressure in the cuff

A false reading

Sometimes a blood pressure measurement can produce false readings that are too high. This happens most often among older adults with damaged arteries that have become very stiff, and it's different from white-coat hypertension (see "Do you have white-coat hypertension" on page 43). Although many people with stiff arteries have increased blood pressure, it may not be as high as measurements indicate.

False readings occur because rigid arteries are difficult to collapse. When a blood pressure measurement is taken, the cuff may not be able to collapse your arm's main (brachial) artery until the cuff has been inflated to a level well above your systolic pressure. And when pressure in the cuff is released, the stiffness causes the artery to open more quickly than it normally should. Therefore, a blood pressure reading doesn't reflect the true pressure inside your arteries.

Your doctor often can tell whether you have this condition, called pseudohypertension, by feeling your forearm. Normally, when a blood pressure cuff collapses your brachial artery, the arteries in your forearm below the cuff also collapse so you can't feel them.

Among people with very stiff arteries, however, vessels in their forearms remain open and can be felt even when no blood is flowing through them. People with this condition may find that electronic sphygmomanometers also fail to give accurate readings.

To get an accurate blood pressure measurement, you may need to have the pressure in your arteries measured by inserting a needle into an artery in your arm.

equals your systolic pressure, blood begins to flow through your artery again. This causes a thumping sound to be heard through the stethoscope. The number on the mercury column or air pressure gauge that coincides with the moment that the return of blood flow is first heard is your systolic pressure.

As air continues to be released from the cuff, pressure on the brachial artery drops further. When the artery is fully open again, the thumping sounds become inaudible. The reading on the mercury column or pressure gauge at the moment the sounds disappear is equivalent to your diastolic pressure (lower number).

Electronic sphygmomanometers work in a similar fashion, but they include a monitor that's fully automatic. It inflates and deflates the cuff, detects your systolic and diastolic pressures and then displays your measurements on a digital screen.

To produce accurate readings, the inflatable part of the cuff needs to cover at least three-quarters of your upper arm. If you will be measuring your own blood pressure, see Chapter 10 for detailed instructions. Also ask your doctor for help.

Making a diagnosis

A blood pressure measurement of 140/90 millimeters of mercury (mm Hg) is considered high. But one reading of 140/90 mm Hg or higher isn't enough for a diagnosis of high blood pressure. Your blood pressure may vary throughout the day, and it's best to obtain multiple readings under similar circumstances. Only if the reading is extremely high — a systolic pressure of 210 mm Hg or higher or a diastolic pressure of 120 mm Hg or higher — is a diagnosis made based on a single measurement.

Generally, a diagnosis of high blood pressure is made only after at least three visits to your doctor. Your blood pressure is measured two or more times at each visit, for a total of at least six measurements. If the average of the six measurements shows your blood pressure to be 140/90 mm Hg or higher, then you have high blood pressure.

If you're older than 65 years, your doctor may take even more measurements before deciding whether you have high blood pressure, because as you get older variations in your blood pressure tend to broaden.

To ensure an accurate reading, it's a good idea not to smoke, eat a big meal or drink caffeine or alcohol for at least 30 minutes before having your blood pressure measured. These factors can all temporarily raise your blood pressure. Also give yourself plenty of time to make it to your appointment. Rushing to an appointment can cause stress, which can also increase your blood pressure temporarily. Before you have your blood pressure measured, sit quietly for a few minutes and

Do you have white-coat hypertension?

Some people — knowingly or unknowingly — become anxious when they have their blood pressure measured. These people may have normal blood pressure at other times, but when it's measured in a medical setting, it's always high. This condition, called white-coat hypertension, is fairly common.

If your doctor suspects your high blood pressure is white-coat hypertension, you may need to measure your blood pressure at home and at work and keep a log of your readings. Or your doctor may recommend that you wear a portable device (ambulatory monitor) that measures your blood pressure periodically over a 24-hour period while you go about your regular activities. These two methods generally give a more realistic and accurate assessment of your blood pressure than does a measurement taken in a medical setting.

Automated machines in stores and shopping malls that measure blood pressure aren't recommended. These machines are usually accurate when first installed, but they can lose their accuracy if they aren't maintained and calibrated regularly.

An important question regarding white-coat hypertension is whether the increase in blood pressure is confined to medical appointments or whether it occurs whenever you feel anxious or stressed. So far, most studies have found the condition to be limited mainly to medical settings. People with white-coat hypertension typically respond to other stress in the same manner as people with normal blood pressure.

Conventional medical thought has been that white-coat hypertension is a harmless phenomenon not requiring treatment. However, some studies suggest the condition may increase your risk of cardiovascular disease and should be carefully monitored and treated. Your doctor may recommend adjustments to your lifestyle, including regular physical activity, improving your diet and reducing stress. He or she may also recommend a blood pressure lowering medication or a medication to control other cardiovascular risk factors.

try to relax. In addition, when having your blood pressure taken, don't talk. Talking makes it harder for the person taking your blood pressure to hear the sound of your heartbeat.

Getting an evaluation

Between the time you first learn that you may have high blood pressure and the time an actual diagnosis is made, your doctor will want to get your medical history, do a physical examination and have you take a few tests.

These three components can provide answers to important questions, such as:

- Has your high blood pressure damaged any of your organs?
- Is your high blood pressure essential or secondary? Although secondary high blood pressure is uncommon, it's important that each person with high blood pressure be considered for secondary causes. Note that some of these causes may be reversible.
- Do you have other risk factors that put you at increased risk of a heart attack or stroke, such as tobacco use, overweight or obesity, an inactive lifestyle, high blood cholesterol or diabetes?

If it's unclear whether you have high blood pressure, these evaluation steps can help confirm the diagnosis.

Medical history

Your medical history may point to a certain factor or event that triggered the increase in your blood pressure. Information from your history can also help your doctor assess your risk of other health conditions.

During an evaluation, you may be asked questions regarding:

- Prior blood pressure readings
- A personal history of heart or kidney problems, high cholesterol, diabetes or restless sleep or daytime sleepiness due to sleep apnea
- A family history of high blood pressure, heart attack, stroke, kidney disease, diabetes, high cholesterol or early (premature) death

- Signs and symptoms suggesting secondary high blood pressure, such as flushing spells, a rapid heart rate, intolerance to heat or unexplained weight loss

You may also be asked questions about your behavior and habits related to:

- Alcohol use
- Tobacco use
- Changes in weight
- Activity level
- Diet and use of salt (sodium)
- Work- or home-related stress
- Medications you're currently taking and previous use of high blood pressure drugs

Be sure to tell your doctor about *all* of the drugs you take — both prescription and over-the-counter (OTC), as well as illicit drugs and alternative products, such as herbal and nutritional supplements.

Several prescription and OTC drugs — including many diet pills, decongestant nasal sprays, cold and allergy medicines, and nonsteroidal anti-inflammatory drugs — can increase your blood pressure. Cocaine and amphetamines also increase blood pressure. Because many alternative supplements haven't been fully studied to determine their health effects, it's important that you tell your doctor if you're taking such a product — just in case it may be increasing your blood pressure.

Some high blood pressure medications don't react well with other drugs. This can lead to problems called drug interactions. Keeping your doctor aware of *all* of the drugs you take can also prevent dangerous interactions should you need to take a blood pressure medication. Keep a list of all medications you take — prescription drugs, OTC drugs and herbal and nutritional products. If you don't have a list, keep all of your medications in their original containers and bring them all to your next doctor visit. For more information about medications, see Chapter 11.

Keep in mind that blood pressure normally rises and falls over any 24-hour period. Diet, daily activities, emotions and other factors can lead to variations in blood pressure. Work with your doctor to set treatment goals that take these variations into account.

Round-the-clock reading

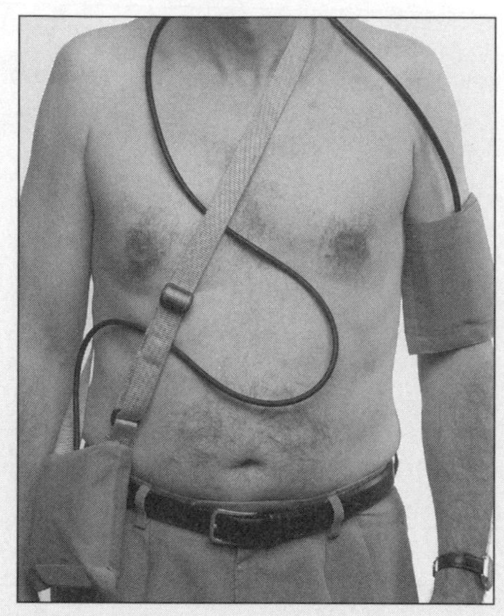

High blood pressure can, at times, be difficult to diagnose. If your doctor is uncertain you have high blood pressure, or is having trouble determining how severe your condition is, you may need to wear an ambulatory monitor.

The procedure involves fitting you with a portable blood pressure device that you wear for a day. It includes an inflatable cuff that fits around your arm and a small monitoring unit that may worn over your shoulder. A thin tube connects the monitor to the cuff. This tube may be secured to your skin with tape to prevent it from disconnecting.

The monitor is programmed to take your blood pressure about every 10 to 30 minutes over 6 to 24 hours. The device is fully automatic. It pumps up the blood pressure cuff, deflates it and stores the reading in its memory.

You may be a candidate for ambulatory monitoring if you have white-coat hypertension — or if you show complications of high blood pressure but have normal blood pressure during medical checkups. Ambulatory monitoring can also be helpful if your blood pressure fluctuates widely or if you're not responding to blood pressure medications. If you're at risk of heart problems or ischemic stroke, your doctor may want you to do electrocardiogram monitoring as well.

Keeping a journal that lists your daily activities and the time you did them, the time you took your medications, and any periods of stress, strong emotion or pain also can be helpful. By matching the journal entries with your blood pressure readings, your doctor can see whether certain events or lifestyle factors may be linked to changes in your blood pressure.

Physical examination

During the physical examination, your doctor will look for signs of organ damage. He or she will also check for abnormalities that might signal a possible cause for the rise in your blood pressure.

Conditions your doctor may check for include:

Narrowed or leaky blood vessels in your eyes. Damage to blood vessels in your eyes is a good indication that blood vessels elsewhere in your body may also be damaged. This damage may also indicate a risk of cardiovascular disease.

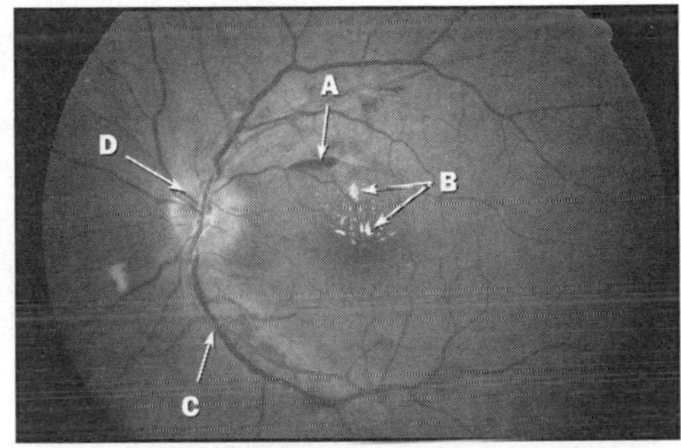

Severe high blood pressure can cause blood vessels in your retina to rupture, causing bleeding (hemorrhaging, see A) and fluid leakage (exudate, see B) in your eye. Narrowing of arteries (see C) and swelling of the optic nerve disk (papillodema, see D) may also occur.

Heart abnormalities. A fast heart rate, an enlarged heart, an abnormal rhythm or a click or murmur can signal possible heart disease.

Turbulent blood flow. When a blood vessel narrows, it can cause turbulent blood flow that can be heard through a stethoscope. The turbulent flow, called a bruit (BRU-we), most often occurs in the carotid arteries in your neck and major arteries in your abdomen.

An aortic aneurysm. It may be felt during examination of your abdomen. A stethoscope also may pick up the sound of blood pulsing through the weakened and bulging blood vessel.

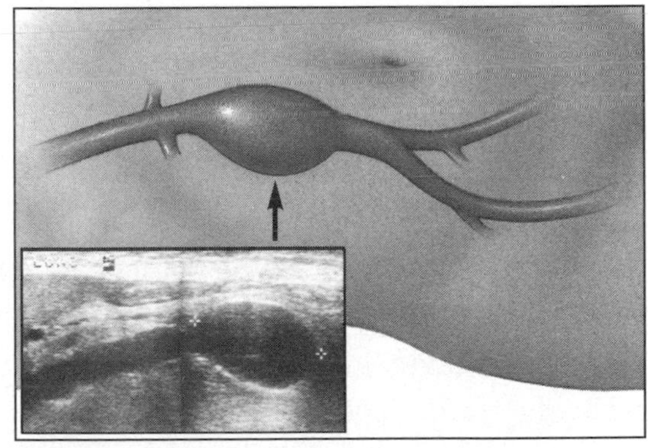
An aortic aneurysm is an expanded region of the aorta (arrow) that may rupture or form a blood clot at the site of expansion. Aneurysms can be viewed and measured with an ultrasound examination (see inset).

Enlarged kidneys or thyroid gland. These are indications that your high blood pressure may be resulting from another condition.

A weakened pulse. A weak pulse in your groin, lower legs and ankles can signal artery damage.

Reduced blood pressure in your ankles. This can result from narrowed or diseased blood vessels in your legs.

Swelling. Accumulation of fluid in your lower legs and ankles is a common sign of heart or kidney failure.

A decrease in blood pressure when you stand. It can help identify if you may be at risk of fainting or dizziness upon standing (postural hypotension), a side effect of some blood pressure medications. Such dizziness is one complication of diabetes. The problem is also common in older adults particularly after meals, whether or not they have diabetes. For more information, see "When your blood pressure drops too low" on page 12.

Routine tests

These tests are commonly part of an evaluation for high blood pressure:

Urinalysis. The presence of protein or red blood cells in your urine can indicate kidney damage. A form of protein in your urine, called microalbuminuria (mi-kro-al-bu-min-U-re-uh), can also signal early-stage kidney disease and is a risk factor for future cardiovascular disease. In addition, your urine may be tested for the presence of sugar (glucose) resulting from diabetes. Diabetes can make high blood pressure more difficult to control.

Blood chemistry. The amounts of sodium and potassium in your blood are measured. Your blood is also tested for levels of certain chemicals, such as creatinine (kre-AT-ih-nin), that can indicate damage to your kidneys.

Other common blood tests include measurement of cholesterol-containing blood fats (lipid profile). The higher your total blood cholesterol level and the lower your level of high-density lipoprotein, or "good," cholesterol, the greater your risk of cardiovascular disease and insulin resistance syndrome. The amount of glucose in your blood also is measured to check for diabetes.

Complete blood cell count. This test determines abnormal white and red blood cell counts. Its purpose is to ensure that you don't have health conditions you may not be aware of, such as a low red blood cell count, called anemia (uh-NE-me-uh).

Electrocardiography. Your heart's electrical activity is recorded to check for abnormalities in its rhythm or for indications of heart enlargement, heart damage or an inadequate supply of blood to your heart muscle.

Changes in your heart's electrical activity as shown on an electrocardiogram (ECG) can also indicate high or low levels of potassium.

Additional tests

If your physical examination and laboratory findings are normal, you probably won't have to have any additional tests. However, further tests may be necessary if you have:

- Sudden onset of high blood pressure or a sharp increase in your usual blood pressure
- Very high blood pressure (180 or higher/110 or higher mm Hg)
- A low blood potassium level
- A bruit over an artery
- Evidence of kidney problems
- Evidence of heart problems
- A possible abdominal aortic aneurysm

If you have narrowed arteries that are interrupting blood flow, these tests can identify the narrowing and its severity:

Angiography. During this procedure, material that makes your arteries visible on X-rays is injected into your arteries and then X-rays are taken of specific vessels.

Magnetic resonance angiography (MRA). This procedure uses energy created by powerful magnets to view arterial blood flow.

Ultrasonography. It uses high-frequency sound waves to show blood flow through an artery. Ultrasonography is also commonly used to identify specific heart and artery abnormalities.

If your doctor suspects you may have a shrunken kidney, an abdominal aortic aneurysm or a tumor, such as an adrenal gland tumor, additional tests may include ultrasonography or:

Computerized tomography (CT). CT scans are three-dimensional X-rays.

Magnetic resonance imaging (MRI). It's similar to MRA, but the scan focuses on organs or regions of the body rather than blood vessels.

Nuclear scanning. It involves injecting radioactive material (radioisotopes) into a vein and then taking nuclear images as the material passes through a specific location or organ. Nuclear scans are used to monitor blood flow, determine the size of an organ or see if an organ is functioning normally.

Deciding on treatment

Treatment of high blood pressure is tailored to your specific needs. That's why the type of treatment that works for someone else may not work for you. How your high blood pressure is treated depends on your blood pressure stage and the results of your medical history, physical examination and laboratory tests. You and your doctor will work together to determine the most effective treatment plan for you.

There are basically two methods for reducing high blood pressure — lifestyle changes and medication. Depending on your health and your risk factors, recommended lifestyle changes may include losing weight, becoming more active, eating a healthier diet, reducing sodium, stopping smoking, limiting alcohol and controlling stress.

Several types of medications are used to control high blood pressure, and there are developments on the horizon. Genetic research indicates that heredity can predict some people's response to drug treatments for high blood pressure. These findings have the potential for better matching individuals with medications to increase the effectiveness of the drugs.

Many types of medications affect your blood pressure in different ways. That's why it's important that you not share high blood pressure pills with anyone. Their medication may not be the same type as yours.

Latest guidelines

The National Heart, Lung, and Blood Institute, a division of the National Institutes of Health, periodically issues a report called the Joint National Committee on Prevention, Detection, Evaluation, and Treatment of High Blood Pressure. The latest report, the sixth, was issued in November 1997 and is often referred to as JNC VI. It divides people with high blood pressure into three risk groups — A, B and C — and makes treatment recommendations for each group. Risk is determined according to blood pressure stage, condition of internal organs, the presence of cardiovascular disease and factors that increase the risk of cardiovascular disease. JNC VI includes recommendations for treating high-normal blood pressure. If you have high-normal blood pressure and don't bring it down to a normal level, there's a good chance it will progress to high blood pressure.

Guidelines from outside the United States — for example, from the World Health Organization-International Society of Hypertension, the British Hypertension Society and the Canadian Hypertension Society — take a similar approach. Recent studies have provided evidence supporting blood pressure goals even lower than those set by these organizations in certain circumstances (see "Setting treatment goals" on page 52).

Risk group A. You're in this risk group if you have high-normal blood pressure or high blood pressure, but you don't have organ damage, cardiovascular disease or other risk factors for cardiovascular disease, such as tobacco use or high cholesterol.

If your blood pressure is in the high-normal range, recommended treatment is lifestyle changes to reduce your blood pressure to a normal or optimal level.

If you have stage 1 high blood pressure, lifestyle changes are also the recommended approach. But if after a year these changes fail to reduce your blood pressure to a normal or optimal level, then you may need medication in addition to lifestyle changes.

If you have stage 2 or stage 3 high blood pressure, initial treatment should include medication in addition to changes in your lifestyle. (See "Guidelines for treatment" on page 53.)

Risk group B. Most people with high blood pressure are in this risk group. It includes people who don't have organ damage or cardiovascular disease but who do have one or more cardiovascular risk factors, excluding diabetes.

If your blood pressure is high-normal, lifestyle changes are recommended. If you have stage 1 high blood pressure, lifestyle changes are the first line of treatment. If after 6 to 12 months lifestyle changes don't reduce your blood pressure, you may need medication. If you have several risk factors, your doctor may prescribe medication right away, in addition to lifestyle changes.

If you have stage 2 or stage 3 high blood pressure, initial treatment should include both lifestyle changes and medication.

Risk group C. This group includes people at greatest risk of heart attack, stroke or other problems related to high blood pressure. You fit into this group if you have cardiovascular disease, organ damage, diabetes or a combination of these.

Medication and changes in lifestyle are the recommended therapy for everyone in this group. Even if your blood pressure is only high-normal, but you have kidney disease, heart failure or diabetes, medication and changes in lifestyle will be required.

Setting treatment goals

Your treatment plan for high blood pressure will include specific goals that take into account your overall health. For example, if you have diabetes or kidney disease or have had a stroke or transient ischemic attack, your blood pressure goal probably will be less than 130/80 mm Hg. This is also a common goal for people who've experienced heart failure. If you have severe kidney disease, a goal of less than 120/75 mm Hg is advised.

Achieving such goals can call for lifestyle changes, medications, or both. Meet with your doctor regularly to review your goals, assess your progress and adjust your treatment plan.

A common misconception

Many people taking high blood pressure medication believe that it's not important to make changes in their lifestyle because their

Guidelines for treatment

Blood pressure stages (mm Hg)	Risk group A	Risk group B	Risk group C
High-normal (130-139/85-89)	Lifestyle changes	Lifestyle changes	Medication* Lifestyle changes
Stage 1 (140-159/90-99)	Lifestyle changes (up to 12 months)	Lifestyle changes† (up to 6 months)	Medication Lifestyle changes
Stages 2 and 3 (≥ 160/≥ 100)	Medication Lifestyle changes	Medication Lifestyle changes	Medication Lifestyle changes

*For people with heart failure, kidney failure or diabetes.

†If you have multiple risk factors, your doctor may consider drugs as initial therapy plus lifestyle changes.

Major risk factors that can affect treatment	Organ damage or disease that can affect treatment
Tobacco use	Heart disease
Undesirable blood fat (lipid) levels	Muscle thickening in main pumping chamber
Diabetes	Previous heart attack or chest pain (angina)
Age (older than 60)	Prior bypass surgery or angioplasty
Sex (male, or post-menopausal female)	Heart failure
Family history of cardiovascular disease	Stroke or transient ischemic attack (ministroke)
	Kidney disease
	Peripheral artery damage
	Retinal damage

Adapted from National Institutes of Health. *The Sixth Report of the Joint National Committee on Prevention, Detection, Evaluation, and Treatment of High Blood Pressure,* 1997.

Numbers on progress are mixed

Since 1972, when the National Heart, Lung, and Blood Institute began an intensive education campaign, there generally has been steady improvement in awareness, treatment and control of high blood pressure. As a result of these gains, death and disability attributed to the disease have declined significantly. Death rates from stroke have dropped by nearly 60 percent, and deaths due to heart attack have declined by more than 50 percent.

But during the 1990s, those dramatic improvements slowed and some of the increases began to reverse. Latest results from the Third National Health and Nutrition Examination Survey (NHANES III, 1991 to 1994) show a small decline in all three categories — high blood pressure awareness, treatment and control. In particular, control rates dropped from 29 percent to 27.4 percent from the previous survey.

The reasons for the recent overall decline are unclear. An increase in obesity and lack of exercise may be factors. In *Health, United States, 2002*, a report by the U.S. Surgeon General, it's noted that three in five adults ages 20 to 74 are overweight, and that one in four Americans is considered to be obese. The report also notes that nearly 40 percent of Americans engage in no physical activity during leisure time.

Another factor may be complacency. Above-normal blood pressures too often may be overlooked — both by doctors and their patients — as being close enough to being in control.

Despite these findings, there is some good news. Recent data gathered on people under age 64 with high blood pressure who received their health care through managed care organizations showed that between 2000 and 2001, there was a 4-percent improvement in blood pressure control rates.

Also in the positive news category are findings that among nearly 6,000 American adults age 65 and older, more were being treated for their high blood pressure in 1999 than were a decade earlier. And more of those being treated reached a goal blood pressure lower than 140/90 millimeters of mercury than did those a decade earlier.

medication is taking care of their problem. That's not true.

Sometimes, medication can reduce your blood pressure by only a certain amount. And that amount may not be enough to bring your blood pressure down to a normal or optimal level. However, lifestyle changes in addition to your medication often can help you reach a normal pressure.

If you're able to achieve a normal blood pressure level with medication, making lifestyle changes may help reduce the amount of medication you need daily. Less medication means less cost. In addition, if your medication causes bothersome side effects, cutting back the dosage may reduce the side effects. A few people who've significantly changed their lifestyle have even been able to stop taking medication entirely.

Finally, lifestyle changes are important for all people with high blood pressure because they can help reduce risk of future health problems, including stroke, heart attack, heart failure, kidney failure and dementia.

Becoming an active partner

It takes a team effort to treat high blood pressure successfully. Your doctor can't do it alone, and neither can you. The two of you need to work together to bring your blood pressure down to a healthy level — and keep it there.

However, even though it's a team effort, you can assume most of the responsibility for controlling your blood pressure. Changing your lifestyle — losing weight, becoming more active and eating a healthier diet — is an important step within your control. Taking medication regularly and properly also is your responsibility, as is knowing the names and doses of all of your medications. So is measuring your blood pressure at home, if that's part of your treatment plan.

You can live a long and healthy life with high blood pressure. But to do that, you need to recognize that high blood pressure is a serious condition and become actively involved in your treatment. For more on controlling your blood pressure, see Chapter 10.

Wrap-up

Key points to remember:

- A diagnosis of high blood pressure generally is made after three separate doctor visits that show persistently high systolic or diastolic pressure, or both.
- A medical history, a physical examination and routine tests are typically part of the process to diagnose high blood pressure.
- Appropriate treatment of high blood pressure depends on blood pressure stage, organ damage, cardiovascular risk factors, diabetes and other diseases.
- The two methods for lowering blood pressure are lifestyle changes and medication.
- Even if you take medication, changes in your lifestyle are essential to controlling high blood pressure.

Chapter 4

Controlling your weight

Your weight and your blood pressure are often closely related. When your weight increases, your blood pressure often does too. As Americans become increasingly overweight, controlling weight has become a major challenge in preventing and controlling high blood pressure. If you're overweight, your risk of developing high blood pressure is two to six times greater than if your weight is healthy. Indeed, 75 percent of cases of high blood pressure in U.S. adults are directly related to obesity.

Just as your blood pressure goes up when you gain weight, it usually goes down when you lose weight. Shedding even a few pounds can bring an improvement in your blood pressure. The most successful method for losing weight is to change your eating and activity habits and slim down slowly.

Doctors recognize that losing weight — and keeping it off — is a difficult task. It takes a lot of effort and willpower to follow a healthy diet and become more physically active. But just because the task may be daunting, it doesn't mean that you shouldn't try — and keep trying. Eventually, your efforts will pay off. For example, researchers found that adults who gained less than 11 pounds after age 18 avoided a variety of weight-related health problems.

Keeping weight off — a problem for many

Studies of individuals at risk of high blood pressure find that maintaining weight loss is difficult for many people. In one large study, only 13 percent of individuals who lost weight were able to maintain their weight loss beyond 3 years. In another study, about 25 percent of participants who lost weight kept it off for 5 years. As their weight crept back up, so did their blood pressure. A similar follow-up study concluded that a low-sodium diet is generally easier for people to maintain than a low-calorie diet. Researchers say that to control high blood pressure, there needs to be greater societal emphasis on controlling obesity through improved diet and increased activity.

Weight and blood pressure

Being overweight doesn't guarantee that you'll have high blood pressure — you can be overweight and have normal blood pressure — but it significantly increases your chances.

A 1998 study involving more than 82,000 women found that women who gained 11 to 22 pounds (5 to 10 kilograms) during adulthood had a 70 percent increase in risk of high blood pressure compared with women who didn't gain weight after age 18. For women who gained more than 22 pounds (10 kilograms), their risk was even higher. Although the study didn't include men, other studies involving men also demonstrate that being overweight increases risk of high blood pressure.

There is good news in all of this. The study also found that losing weight decreases your risk. Overweight women who lost 11 to 22 pounds (5 to 10 kilograms) lowered their risk by 15 percent. And women who lost more than 22 pounds (10 kilograms) cut their risk by more than 25 percent.

What's the link between body weight and high blood pressure? As you put on weight, you gain mostly fatty tissue. Just like other parts of your body, this tissue relies on oxygen and nutrients in your blood to survive. As demand for oxygen and nutrients increases, the amount of blood circulating through your body also increases. More blood traveling through your arteries means added pressure on your artery walls.

Another reason blood pressure commonly rises in overweight individuals is that additional weight typically increases the level of insulin in blood. Increased insulin is associated with retention of sodium and water, which raises blood volume. In addition, excess weight can increase your heart rate and reduce the capacity of your blood vessels to transport blood. These two factors also can raise blood pressure.

Recently, a number of hormones, including leptin and ghrelin, have been identified. These hormones interact with each other and with insulin, and they influence appetite, weight and blood pressure. The role of these hormones is being studied to determine how they work and how they affect weight control and the treatment of high blood pressure.

If you're at risk of high blood pressure, weight loss may prevent its development. If you already have high blood pressure, losing weight may prevent the need for medication. If you're already taking medication, weight loss can help control your blood pressure and possibly reduce how much medication you need each day — or perhaps even eliminate your need for medication. However, even though you may no longer be taking medication, you're still at risk of high blood pressure recurring. Therefore, you need to monitor your weight and blood pressure regularly.

Just a little can mean a lot

You don't have to lose a large amount of weight to lower your blood pressure. Losing as little as 10 pounds (4.5 kilograms) can reduce blood pressure. And when you lose as little as 10 percent of your weight, you may reduce your blood pressure to a healthier level. Shedding a few pounds can also improve your cholesterol levels and reduce your risk of heart attack, stroke, diabetes and arthritis.

If you're overweight, reducing your weight by 10 percent may be a good goal. Once you've achieved that goal, you can try for another 10 percent if you need to lose more weight. Over a few years, these losses can add up to a significant improvement in your weight and health.

Overweight vs. obesity

According to 2002 government surveys, nearly 65 percent of American adults are overweight and of that group, nearly half — about 31 percent — are obese. During the past few decades, the entire U.S. population has gotten heavier and the percentage of people who are obese has almost doubled.

In addition to contributing to higher blood pressure, the degree to which you're overweight contributes to your risk of other health problems. Obesity significantly increases your risk of diabetes, heart disease, stroke, arthritis and some cancers. The difference between being overweight and obese is a matter of degree. Health care guidelines define overweight as having a body mass index (BMI) of 25 to 29.9. Obesity refers to a BMI of 30 or more.

Body mass index is a formula that factors in your weight and your height in determining whether you have a healthy or unhealthy percentage of total body fat. Except in very muscular people, this measurement correlates well with total body fat. It's a better measurement of health risks related to your weight than is using your bathroom scale or standard weight-and-height tables. Unlike weight-and-height tables, body mass index doesn't differentiate between men and women.

To determine your BMI, locate your height on the chart on the next page and follow it across until you reach the weight nearest yours. Look at the top of the column for the BMI rating. If your weight is less than the weight nearest yours, your BMI may be slightly less. If your weight is greater than the weight nearest yours, your BMI may be slightly greater. A BMI of 18.5 to 24.9 is considered healthy. A BMI of 25 to 29.9 signifies overweight, and a BMI of 30 or more indicates obesity.

You can also calculate your BMI by using this formula:

Step 1. Multiply your weight in pounds by 0.45.

Step 2. Multiply your height in inches by 0.0254.

Step 3. Square your answer from step 2.

Step 4. Divide your answer from step 1 by your answer from step 3.

The resulting answer is your BMI.

What's your BMI?

Body mass index (BMI)

	Healthy		Overweight					Obesity				
BMI	**19**	**24**	25	26	27	28	29	30	35	40	45	50
Height			Weight in pounds									
4′10″	91	115	119	124	129	134	138	143	167	191	215	239
4′11″	94	119	124	128	133	138	143	148	173	198	222	247
5′0″	97	123	128	133	138	143	148	153	179	204	230	255
5′1″	100	127	132	137	143	148	153	158	185	211	238	264
5′2″	104	131	136	142	147	153	158	164	191	218	246	273
5′3″	107	135	141	146	152	158	163	169	197	225	254	282
5′4″	110	140	145	151	157	163	169	174	204	232	262	291
5′5″	114	144	150	156	162	168	174	180	210	240	270	300
5′6″	118	148	155	161	167	173	179	186	216	247	278	309
5′7″	121	153	159	166	172	178	185	191	223	255	287	319
5′8″	125	158	164	171	177	184	190	197	230	262	295	328
5′9″	128	162	169	176	182	189	196	203	236	270	304	338
5′10″	132	167	174	181	188	195	202	209	243	278	313	348
5′11″	136	172	179	186	193	200	208	215	250	286	322	358
6′0″	140	177	184	191	199	206	213	221	258	294	331	368
6′1″	144	182	189	197	204	212	219	227	265	302	340	378
6′2″	148	186	194	202	210	218	225	233	272	311	350	389
6′3″	152	192	200	208	216	224	232	240	279	319	359	399
6′4″	156	197	205	213	221	230	238	246	287	328	369	410

Adapted from *Clinical Guidelines on the Identification, Evaluation, and Treatment of Overweight and Obesity in Adults*, 1998.

If you're using the metric system, your BMI equals your weight in kilograms divided by the square of your height in meters.

For an example, see "BMI worksheet" below.

BMI worksheet

Example BMI: BMI for person who is 5 feet, 6 inches tall (66 inches) and weighs 160 pounds	**Your BMI:** Now use your own weight and height to calculate your BMI
Step 1: 160 x 0.45 = 72	**Step 1:** ________ x 0.45 = ________ (your weight in pounds)
Step 2: 66 x 0.0254 = 1.68	**Step 2:** ________ x 0.0254 = ________ (your height in inches)
Step 3: 1.68 x 1.68 = 2.82	**Step 3:** ________ x ________ = ________ (step 2 answer) (step 2 answer)
Step 4: 72 divided by 2.82 = 25.5	**Step 4:** ________ ÷ ________ = ________ (step 1 answer) (step 3 answer) (your BMI)
This person's estimated BMI is 25.5	

Finding your healthy weight

What is a healthy weight? If you have high blood pressure, or if you're at risk, it's not critical that you become thin. But you can try to achieve or maintain a weight that improves control of your blood pressure and also lessens your risks of other health problems.

The three do-it-yourself evaluations that follow can tell you whether your weight is healthy or whether you could benefit from losing a few pounds.

Body mass index

The first step in determining your healthy weight is to figure out your body mass index (BMI). You can determine your BMI by using the BMI chart on page 61 or the formula above.

You're at increased risk of developing a weight-related disease, such as high blood pressure, if your BMI is 25 or greater.

Fat factors

Eating too much and exercising too little are most often responsible for weight gain. When you eat more calories than you use, you store them as fat. However, overeating and inactivity aren't always the problem. Other factors can influence your weight:

Your genes. Heredity doesn't automatically mean you'll be fat, but your genes can make you more susceptible to weight gain. They affect the rate at which your body accumulates fat and where your fat is stored. A family history of obesity increases your chances of becoming obese by about 25 percent to 30 percent. For example, a study in Great Britain found that boys were eight times more likely to be obese if both parents were obese.

Other obesity risk factors, such as the foods you eat and your activity habits, are strongly influenced by your family as well.

Your sex. Men generally have a metabolic rate 5 percent to 10 percent higher than that of women and can often eat more than women without gaining weight. Men also use an average of 10 percent to 20 percent more calories than do women during exercise.

Your age. As you get older, the amount of muscle in your body tends to decrease. As a result, your metabolism slows. This reduces your need for calories. Eating the same amounts of food you ate when you were younger can lead to weight gain — often adding an extra pound a year after age 35.

A high-calorie diet. Pay attention to portion sizes. Larger portions mean more calories. Consuming just 10 calories more than you burn each day can add 2 pounds of body fat a year. Multiply that by 30 years, and it's easy to see why so many Americans are overweight.

Many people mistakenly assume that all foods low in fat are also low in calories. Consuming foods and beverages that are calorie dense, or high in calories — even though they may be low in fat — also can result in weight gain.

Medical problems. Less than 2 percent of all cases of obesity can be traced to a health condition, such as a metabolic disorder or a hormonal imbalance. However, some medications, including some oral steroids and antidepressants, commonly lead to weight gain.

Waist circumference

This measurement — used in combination with your BMI — is also important in evaluating healthy weight. It indicates where most of your fat is located. Within the BMI categories, fat accumulation around your waist — as well as within your abdomen — is associated with an increased risk of high blood pressure, in addition to other diseases such as diabetes, abnormal cholesterol levels, insulin resistance syndrome, coronary artery disease, stroke and certain types of cancer.

To determine whether you're carrying too much weight around your abdomen, measure your waist circumference. Find the highest point on each of your hip bones and measure across your abdomen just above those highest points. A measurement of more than 40 inches (102 centimeters) in men and 35 inches (88 centimeters) in women signifies increased health risks, especially if you have a BMI of 25 or more.

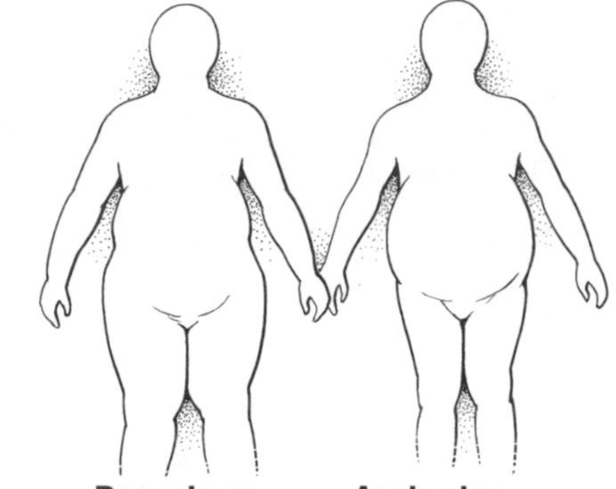

It's not only how much you weigh that's important but also where your body stores extra fat. For two people with the same body mass index, the person with more of an apple shape has a higher risk of health problems than does the person who has more of a pear shape.

Personal and family history

Numbers alone aren't enough. An evaluation of your personal medical history, along with that of your family's, is equally important for determining whether your weight is healthy.

Answer these questions:

- Do you have a health condition, such as high blood pressure, diabetes, high cholesterol or arthritis?
- Do you have a family history of a weight-related illness, such as type 2 diabetes (formerly called adult-onset or noninsulin-dependent diabetes), high blood pressure, high cholesterol, high triglycerides or sleep apnea?
- Have you gained considerable weight since high school? Weight gain in adulthood is associated with increased health risks.

- Do you smoke cigarettes, have more than two alcoholic drinks a day if you're a man and more than one drink a day if you're a woman, or live with significant stress?

In combination with these factors, excess weight can have greater health implications.

Adding up the results

If your BMI shows that you aren't overweight and you're not carrying too much weight around your abdomen, there's probably no health advantage to changing your weight. Your weight is healthy.

If your BMI is between 25 and 29.9, you may benefit from losing a few pounds, particularly if your waist circumference equals or exceeds healthy guidelines or you answered yes to at least one personal and family health question. Discuss your weight with your doctor during your next checkup.

If your BMI is 30 or more, losing some weight will improve your health and reduce your risk of future illness.

Steps to successful weight loss

If your BMI is too high and you need to lose weight, here are some steps to help you lose weight safely and keep it off permanently. As any veteran dieter knows, losing weight is difficult to do. And it's even more difficult to keep the weight off. But keep trying. Maintaining a healthy weight takes effort.

Many products and programs promise to help you shed pounds. However, the best way to reduce your BMI and improve your blood pressure is through lifestyle changes:

Make a commitment. You must be motivated to lose weight because it's what you want, not what someone else wants you to do.

Only you can help yourself lose weight. However, that doesn't mean that you have to do everything alone. Your doctor, a registered dietitian or other health care professional can help you develop a plan to lose weight. And don't be afraid to ask for support from your spouse, family and friends.

Think positively. Don't dwell on what you're giving up to lose weight. Concentrate instead on the progress you're making.

Commercial weight-loss programs

Many people trying to lose weight find that doing it with others is easier. That's why millions of Americans enroll in commercial weight-loss programs each year. These programs can be helpful, but not all of them approach weight loss in a manner that's safe and effective.

Before you enroll, make sure the program meets the following five criteria:

Safety. The program should ensure that you get adequate nutrition. Although diets may be low in calories, they should still provide the daily recommended amounts of nutrients without the need for unusual supplements or special foods.

Reasonable weight goals. Some people with certain health conditions may benefit from rapid weight loss. But in general, weight loss should be slow and steady. Rapid weight loss is mainly loss of fluid, not fat. Look for a program that's geared toward helping you lose 1 to 2 pounds (0.5 or 1 kilogram) a week. Remember: A loss of just 10 pounds (4.5 kilograms) can have a positive effect on your blood pressure.

Physician participation. The program should encourage consultation with your doctor. Talk with your doctor if you plan to go on a very-low-calorie diet. If you have health problems or you regularly take medication, check with your doctor before taking part in a weight-loss plan.

Attention to permanent lifestyle changes. Losing weight does little good if you don't keep it off. The program should also help you improve your lifelong exercise and eating habits so that you can maintain a healthy weight.

Upfront costs. Know exactly how much the program, including regular follow-up, will cost you.

Rather than thinking, "I really miss eating a doughnut at breakfast," tell yourself, "I feel a lot better when I eat whole-wheat toast and cereal in the morning."

Get your priorities straight. Timing is critical. Don't try to lose weight if you're distracted by other major problems. Chances are, you'll only be setting yourself up for failure.

It takes a lot of mental and physical energy to change habits.

If you're having family or financial problems or you're unhappy with other major aspects of your life, you may be less able to follow through on your good intentions.

Set a realistic goal. Don't try to reach a weight that meets social ideals for thinness but is unrealistic. Instead, aim for a weight that improves your blood pressure, blood sugar and blood cholesterol levels. Check your blood pressure weekly — it often responds more quickly to healthy changes in diet than the scale does — and recognize that healthy weight loss is slow and steady. It's worth repeating that a good weight-loss plan generally involves losing no more than 1 to 2 pounds a week. Set weekly or monthly goals that allow you to check off your successes.

Know your habits. To become aware of your eating behavior, ask yourself if you tend to eat when you're bored, angry, tired, anxious, depressed or socially pressured. If you do, try these possible solutions:

- Before eating anything, ask yourself if you really want it.
- Learn to say no and stay committed.
- Do something to distract yourself from your desire to eat, such as telephone a friend or run an errand.
- If you're feeling stressed or you're angry, direct that energy constructively. This is a good time for a brisk, 30-minute walk or to clean your closet or the garage.

If you have trouble identifying emotions or situations that cause you to eat, try keeping a notebook. List what, when and why you eat. See if any relationships or patterns emerge.

Change gradually. When you've identified problem behaviors that you'd like to change, remember that gradual changes work best. Choose one area at a time, and be specific about how you're going to improve that behavior. When you've successfully changed one habit, work on another. Continually practice your new behaviors so that they become habits.

Plan ahead. Your old habits may be so ingrained that you do them instinctively. Mentally rehearsing new habits can help. Imagine yourself at a party overflowing with rich hors d'oeuvres or fancy desserts. Envision yourself taking a small portion of a few items and leaving space between them on your plate. Mentally rehearse this plan until you feel you can remember it and do it.

In addition, remember that drinking alcohol can affect self-control and the amount that you drink may affect how well you stick to your plan for managing calories.

In the past, you may have told yourself that you deserve certain high-calorie or high-fat foods as a way to reward yourself or relieve stress. Instead, take another approach. Tell yourself that you may deserve it but you don't need it.

To reinforce this idea, visualize the effect of a fattening entree or dessert on your body. In your mind's eye, see the food turning directly into a moist layer of yellow, wiggly fat around your waist. Holding that mental picture can help you deal with food temptation.

Don't starve yourself. Extremely low-calorie diets and special food combinations aren't the answer to long-term weight control and better health. Four national surveys found that most people try to lose weight by eating 1,000 to 1,500 calories a day. However, cutting calories to fewer than 1,200 if you're a woman or 1,400 if you're a man doesn't provide enough food to keep you satisfied, and you get hungry before your next meal. See "Calculating calories" below to determine your calorie needs.

Eating fewer than 1,200 calories also makes it difficult to get adequate amounts of certain nutrients, such as folic acid, magnesium and zinc. In addition, it promotes temporary loss of fluids and loss of healthy muscle rather than permanent loss of fat.

Over-the-counter appetite suppressants also aren't recommended if you're trying to lose weight because they contain adrenaline-like

Calculating calories

Here's an easy way to figure out how many calories you can eat a day and still lose an average of 1 pound (0.5 kilogram) a week:

________________ x 10 = __________
(current weight in pounds) (daily calories)

or

________________ x 22 = __________
(current weight in kilograms) (daily calories)

Use this calorie level as your daily target.

substances that can increase your blood pressure. Of particular concern are products containing ephedra, a dietary supplement touted for its weight-loss characteristics. Ephedra has been associated with a variety of serious health problems and should be avoided.

The best way for most people to lose weight is to eat nutritious foods and change their eating habits. Cut back on total calories by eating nutrient-rich foods such as whole grains, fruits and vegetables. Eat high-calorie foods sparingly. Healthy eating is discussed in more detail in Chapter 6.

Get and stay active. Dieting alone will help you lose weight. But by adding a 30-minute brisk walk most days of the week, you can increase your rate of weight loss. Physical activity is the most important factor related to long-term weight loss. It promotes loss of body fat and development of muscle. These changes in body composition help raise the rate at which you burn calories, making it easier to maintain your weight loss.

Aim for at least 30 minutes of moderate activity on most, if not all, days of the week. Contrary to some people's beliefs, physical activity doesn't have to be strenuous or unenjoyable. See Chapter 7 for more about activities that can help you lose weight.

Consider medical treatments. If a 6 month trial including diet, exercise and behavior change isn't successful in helping you lose weight and your BMI is greater than 27, your doctor may prescribe sibutramine (Meridia). Sibutramine is designed to enhance the feeling of fullness (satiety) and make it easier for you to feel satisfied while eating less. Sibutramine may increase your blood pressure and heart rate. It's not recommended for people with coronary artery disease.

Another weight-loss drug is orlistat (Xenical). It acts by interfering with fat absorption in your digestive system, preventing your body from incorporating some of the calories it would otherwise take on as fat. Orlistat can cause frequent, loose stools.

If you have a BMI between 35 and 40, your doctor may suggest gastric bypass surgery. In this procedure, a portion of your stomach or small intestine may be removed or bypassed so that you need less food.

Maintain your progress. Don't let setbacks weaken your commitment to lose weight. Practice habit changes. Rethink what you can do put the healthy habit back into your daily routine so that you'll succeed next time. Perfection isn't important — persistence is.

Think lifelong. Incorporate healthy behaviors into your life. A few days or weeks is only practice. Researchers are learning more about how genetics and your body contribute to the development of obesity. This information may lead to improved treatments for obesity. However, healthy eating and exercise will likely always be important in maintaining a healthy weight.

Wrap-up

Key points to remember:

- The number of Americans who are overweight or obese continues to increase.
- Your risk of high blood pressure is increased if you've gained more than 10 pounds (4.5 kilograms) as an adult.
- Blood pressure generally increases with weight gain and decreases with weight loss.
- Losing as few as 10 pounds (4.5 kilograms) can lower your blood pressure.
- Be realistic. Aim for a healthy weight.
- Slow, steady weight loss based on eating nutritious foods and getting regular physical activity is the best approach.
- Good weight-loss programs stress a gradual loss of weight and lifestyle changes in diet and exercise. If you still have trouble losing weight or maintaining weight loss, ask your doctor about medical treatments such as medications or surgery.

Chapter 5

The shakedown on salt

Of all the issues related to high blood pressure, none has been more debated than salt — more specifically, the sodium in salt. Despite the controversy, results of studies continue to support the fact that limiting sodium intake — especially if you have high blood pressure — is good for you. Regardless of race, age or sex, the evidence is clear that, in many cases, high blood pressure can be lowered by reducing sodium intake with no adverse effects. (See "DASH-Sodium and TONE studies" on page 74.)

In this chapter, you'll learn how sodium can affect blood pressure and why controlling sodium intake can help you manage high blood pressure. You'll also discover why avoiding excessive sodium is reasonable and safe.

Sodium's role

Sodium is an essential mineral. Its main role is to help maintain the right balance of fluids in your body. It also helps transmit nerve impulses that influence contraction and relaxation of your muscles.

You get sodium from the foods you eat. Many foods naturally contain some sodium. However, most sodium comes from compounds added to food during commercial processing and meal

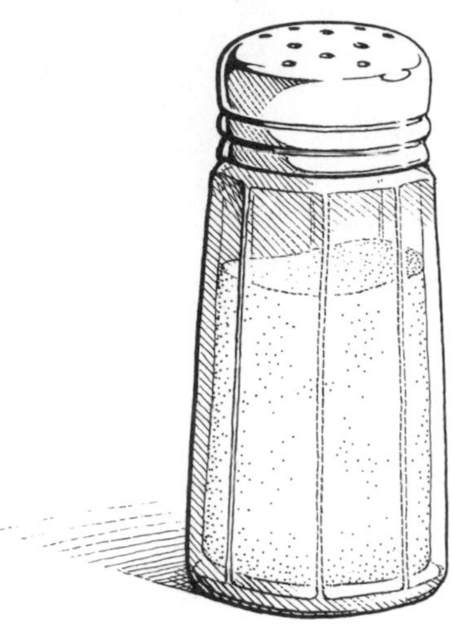

Sodium sources
1% drinking water
11% table and cooking salt
11% naturally inherent in food
77% processed foods

preparation at home. Salt (sodium chloride) is the most common source of sodium. It's made up of 40 percent sodium and 60 percent chloride.

You need only about 500 milligrams (mg) of sodium each day. That's a little more than what's found in ¼ teaspoon of salt. However, it's estimated that the average daily intake for individuals in the United States is between 4,000 and 6,000 mg of sodium.

Your kidneys regulate the amount of sodium in your body. When your sodium levels are low, your kidneys conserve sodium. When your levels are high, they excrete the excess amount in your urine.

Sometimes, though, your kidneys can't eliminate enough sodium and it starts to accumulate in your blood. Because sodium attracts and holds water, your blood volume increases. Your heart has to work harder to move the increased volume of blood through your blood vessels, increasing pressure on your arteries. Heart, kidney, liver and lung diseases all can lead to an inability to regulate sodium. In addition, some people are simply more sensitive to sodium.

Sodium sensitivity

How people react to sodium varies. Some people — both healthy adults and people with high blood pressure — can consume as much sodium as they like, and it has little or no effect on their blood pressure.

For others, too much sodium quickly leads to an increase in blood pressure, often triggering the development of high blood pressure. This condition is referred to as sodium or salt sensitivity.

Approximately 60 percent of Americans with high blood pressure and 25 percent of Americans with normal blood pressure are

Sodium-based food additives

These sodium compounds are commonly added to food during processing and cooking.

Salt (sodium chloride). Used in cooking or at the table; used in canning and preserving.

Monosodium glutamate (MSG). A flavor enhancer used in home and restaurant cooking and in many packaged, canned and frozen foods.

Baking soda (sodium bicarbonate). Sometimes used to leaven breads and cakes; sometimes added to vegetables in cooking; used as an alkalizer for indigestion.

Baking powder. A mixture of baking soda, starch and an acid used to leaven quick breads and cakes.

Disodium phosphate. Present in some quick-cooking cereals and processed cheeses.

Sodium alginate. Used in many chocolate milks and ice creams to make a smooth mixture.

Sodium benzoate. Used as a preservative in many condiments, such as relishes, sauces and salad dressings.

Sodium hydroxide. Used in food processing to soften and loosen skins of ripe olives and certain fruits and vegetables.

Sodium nitrate. Used in cured meats and sausages.

Sodium propionate. Used in pasteurized cheese and in some breads and cakes to inhibit growth of molds.

Sodium sulfite. Used to bleach certain fruits, such as maraschino cherries and glazed or crystallized fruits that are to be artificially colored; used as a preservative in some dried fruits, such as prunes.

Source: American Heart Association, *Sodium and Blood Pressure,* © 1996. Reprinted with permission.

sodium sensitive. The condition is more common in blacks and adults age 65 and older. In addition, people with diabetes tend to be more sensitive to high levels of sodium. Exactly what causes sodium sensitivity isn't known. Genetics may play a role in some cases, especially among blacks.

There's no easy way to tell if you're sodium sensitive, other than to limit sodium in your diet. If you have a sensitivity to sodium, a low-sodium diet should produce a noticeable reduction in your blood pressure. Medical tests can pinpoint your response to varying levels of sodium, but testing isn't practical or necessary.

Reducing sodium is important for another reason. A study published in 2001 found that sodium sensitivity increases your risk of death, whether or not you have high blood pressure. Participants in this study who were sodium sensitive had a higher death rate due to heart disease and other health-related causes than did people who weren't sodium sensitive. In addition to increasing your blood pressure, sensitivity to sodium can increase your risk of kidney problems and left ventricular hypertrophy, a condition in which your heart's main pumping chamber enlarges and doesn't function properly.

If you have high blood pressure, your doctor may recommend a diuretic medication to reduce excess sodium and fluid in your body. A diuretic medication can enhance the effectiveness of other blood pressure lowering medications.

Even if you take a diuretic, it's still important to reduce sodium in your diet. Too much sodium can reduce the blood pressure lowering effect of the diuretic medication you're taking. In addition, making sure you get enough potassium will further help to control your sodium levels.

DASH-Sodium and TONE studies

The 1997 Dietary Approaches to Stop Hypertension (DASH) study demonstrated that a diet rich in fruits, vegetables, grains and low-fat dairy products reduces blood pressure. But some important questions remained. What happens when you combine a healthy diet with reduced sodium? Will the combination reduce blood pressure any further? A follow-up study, called the DASH-Sodium study, as well as a separate study (TONE), provided the answers.

Results of the DASH-Sodium study were published in January 2001. They showed that no matter what your diet, reducing sodium reduces blood pressure. However, the greatest reduction in blood pressure occurs when you combine reduced sodium intake with a healthy diet.

In the study, researchers assigned 412 people to either the DASH diet or a typical American diet, which tends to be higher in fat and lower in fruits, vegetables and grains. Participants ate the assigned diet for 30 days at each of three levels — 3,300 mg, 2,400 mg and 1,500 mg — of sodium intake. The three levels represented high-sodium, moderate-sodium and low-sodium consumption.

In both types of diets, a decrease in blood pressure was observed with lower sodium consumption. The greatest reductions in blood pressure occurred in participants on the DASH diet who kept sodium intake below 1,500 mg a day. Among people who ate the DASH diet at the lowest sodium level, their average systolic blood pressure reading was 11.5 millimeters of mercury (mm Hg) lower than that of participants who ate the standard American diet at the highest sodium level. Even among people who didn't have high blood pressure, the DASH and low-sodium combination resulted in an average drop of 7.1 mm Hg in systolic pressure.

Researchers concluded that in addition to controlling high blood pressure, a healthy diet that's lower in sodium can help prevent the condition. However, researchers acknowledged that limiting sodium consumption to 1,500 mg daily may be a challenge for some people, given the amount of sodium in many processed foods. For help with planning low-sodium meals, see "Menus with DASH" on page 191.

The Trial of Nonpharmacologic Interventions in the Elderly (TONE) study involved 681 participants ages 60 to 80 years and was published in 1998. It also provides strong evidence that reducing dietary sodium lowers blood pressure in sodium-sensitive people and that you're never too old to benefit. In the TONE study, researchers placed participants — all of whom had their blood pressure under control with one anti-hypertensive medication — in one of four groups. One group went on a reduced-sodium diet, another group was put on a weight-loss diet, a third group went on a combined reduced-sodium and weight-loss diet, and the fourth (control) group maintained its regular diet. After 3 months, all blood pressure medications were withdrawn. Participants were then followed from 12 to 32 months to see how long it took before they would again need medication to control their blood pressure. At the end of the follow-up, 43 percent of participants in the combined weight-loss and low-sodium group were still off medication, and 38 percent of the low-sodium-only group still didn't require medication. That compared with 36 percent in the weight-loss-only group and just 25 percent in the control group who didn't require medication to control their blood pressure. Researchers concluded that reduced sodium intake alone, or combined with weight loss, can effectively control high blood pressure. There was no evidence that reduced sodium intake resulted in any cardiovascular problems.

Current recommendation

Much of what you eat, especially processed foods, contains far more sodium than you need. It's estimated that about 90 percent of your sodium intake is from the foods you eat and only about 10 percent from salt you add in cooking or at the table.

The National High Blood Pressure Education Program, sponsored by the National Institutes of Health, recommends that all Americans limit sodium to less than 2,400 mg a day. That's equivalent to what's contained in about a teaspoon of salt. However, the DASH-Sodium and TONE studies confirm that even lower sodium consumption is better.

Many health professionals and organizations, including doctors in Mayo Clinic's Division of Hypertension, support a reduced-sodium diet. Here's why:

- If you have high blood pressure, reducing sodium can lower your blood pressure. Limiting sodium in combination with making other lifestyle changes may be enough to keep you from having to take medication to control your blood pressure.

- If you're taking blood pressure medication, limiting sodium can help increase the effectiveness of the drug.
- If you're at risk of high blood pressure, limiting sodium and making other lifestyle changes may prevent its development.
- If you're healthy, limiting sodium as part of a healthy diet is safe and reasonable. In addition, it may keep you from increased risk of the disease as you get older, when high blood pressure is more prevalent and sensitivity to sodium often increases.

Although doctors can't predict that reducing sodium will reduce your lifetime risk of high blood pressure, large population studies show that when people consume less sodium, their blood pressures are lower. There are also fewer deaths from heart attack and stroke in such groups.

The controversy

Since the recommendation 30 years ago that all Americans — not just those with high blood pressure — limit sodium, it has been a source of some controversy. It's true that when some people with normal blood pressure cut back on sodium, their blood pressure decreases very little, if at all. However, it's also true that for a large population, even a small reduction in average blood pressure — perhaps just 2 mm Hg — can mean significant positive outcomes for the overall health of that population.

Also contributing to the debate are studies suggesting that losing weight and eating a diet that emphasizes grains, fruits, vegetables and low-fat dairy products — or a combination of this diet with low-sodium intake — are more effective in managing high blood pressure than limiting sodium alone. In addition, a 1998 study published in the medical journal *The Lancet* found that participants in the First National Health and Nutrition Examination Survey (NHANES I, 1971 to 1975) who reported eating very little sodium had more heart attacks years later than did those who consumed more sodium. The scientific method used in 1998 study has been questioned.

Making sense of sodium labeling

You'll find sodium-related terms on many foods. Here's what they mean:

Sodium-free or salt-free. Each serving contains less than 5 milligrams (mg) of sodium.

Very low sodium. Each serving contains 35 mg of sodium or less.

Low sodium. Each serving contains 140 mg of sodium or less.

Reduced or less sodium. The product contains at least 25 percent less sodium than the regular version.

Lite or light in sodium. The sodium content has been reduced by at least 50 percent from the regular version.

Unsalted or no salt added. No salt is added during processing of a food that normally contains salt. However, some foods with these labels may still be high in sodium.

Officials with the National High Blood Pressure Education Program continue to monitor scientific information about sodium and blood pressure. Their position is that the bulk of the evidence continues to suggest that avoiding sodium is reasonable and safe. They also believe that for people who are sodium sensitive, sodium control is especially important. In addition, although restricting sodium may benefit some individuals only minimally, for the nation as a whole, it can have a major effect in terms of preventing future high blood pressure and reducing death and disability due to related strokes, heart attacks and heart failure. Overweight people in particular experience a greater number of cardiovascular problems related to higher sodium intake.

What you should do

If your doctor or a registered dietitian has suggested that you cut back on sodium to lower your blood pressure, it's advice you should follow. Even if you haven't been told to reduce sodium, try to limit the amount you eat each day.

There are several ways you can do this:

Eat more fresh and fewer processed foods. Fresh foods usually have less sodium than processed ones. Most fresh fruits and vegetables are naturally low in sodium. Canned vegetables and vegetable juices, such as tomato juice, usually have added salt.

Fresh meat is lower in sodium than luncheon meat, bacon, hot dogs, sausage and ham. All of these foods have sodium added to flavor and help preserve them. However, some fresh meats have salt injected and may be labeled, "Flavor enhanced with saline solution." Check the Nutrition Facts label and avoid meats with more than 200 mg of sodium per serving.

Soups, frozen dinners, sauces, mixes and many other instant products typically have added salt. Snacks such as potato chips, corn chips, pretzels, popcorn, crackers and nuts often have a large amount of added salt. It's best to eat them sparingly.

Chose lower-sodium products. Some processed foods that are high in sodium are also prepared in lower-sodium versions. These include soups, broths, canned vegetables and vegetable juices, processed lean meats, ketchup and soy sauce. Just because a food is low in fat or calories doesn't mean it's low in sodium. Sometimes extra sodium is added to low-fat products to enhance flavor.

Read labels. The Nutrition Facts label tells you how much sodium is in each serving. It also lists whether salt or sodium-containing compounds are ingredients. If sodium is one of the first three ingredients listed, the product is high in sodium. Look for other sources of sodium, such as monosodium glutamate (MSG), baking soda or baking powder.

Some over-the-counter medications also contain large amounts of sodium. They include some antacids, alkalizers (Alka-Seltzer, Bromo Seltzer), laxatives and cough medicines. If you use such a product frequently, check the label or ask your pharmacist to find out its sodium content.

Don't add salt to food when cooking. Remove salt from recipes whenever possible. Cook rice, pasta and hot cereals without adding salt. A dash of salt contains ⅛ teaspoon (300 mg) of sodium.

Don't add salt at the table. If you think your food needs more flavor, try another seasoning, such as lemon, pepper or a sodium-free herb blend.

Spice it up

It's easy to make food taste good without using salt. Here are suggestions for herbs, spices and flavorings you can use to enhance the flavor of certain foods. Tip: Place dried herbs in a little liquid a few minutes before adding to a recipe to help release flavors.

Meat, poultry, fish	
Beef	Bay leaf, dry mustard, marjoram, nutmeg, onion, pepper, sage, thyme
Chicken	Dill, ginger, oregano, paprika, parsley, rosemary, sage, tarragon, thyme
Fish	Bay leaf, curry powder, dry mustard, lemon juice, paprika
Lamb	Cranberry, curry powder, garlic, rosemary
Pork	Cranberry, garlic, onion, oregano, pepper, sage
Veal	Bay leaf, curry powder, ginger, oregano
Vegetables	
Broccoli	Lemon juice, oregano
Carrots	Cinnamon, honey, nutmeg, rosemary, sage
Cauliflower	Nutmeg, tarragon
Corn	Chives, cumin, fresh tomatoes, green pepper, paprika, parsley
Green beans	Dill, lemon juice, nutmeg, tarragon, unsalted French dressing
Peas	Mint, onion, parsley
Potatoes	Dill, garlic, green pepper, onion, parsley, sage
Tomatoes	Basil, dill, onion, oregano, parsley, sage
Low-sodium soups	
Creamed	Bay leaf, dill, paprika, peppercorns, tarragon
Vegetable	Basil, bay leaf, curry, dill, garlic, onion, oregano
Other	
Popcorn	Curry, garlic powder, onion powder
Rice	Basil, cumin, curry, green pepper, oregano
Salads	Basil, dill, lemon juice, parsley, vinegar

Limit your use of condiments. Salad dressings, sauces, dips, ketchup, mustard and relish all contain sodium. Pickles and olives contain a very high amount of sodium.

Rinse canned foods. Rinsing canned vegetables and meats helps remove some of the sodium, but don't rely on this as a way to reduce sodium. It only removes about one-third of the sodium.

Kosher meats. To kosher meat without using salt, broil the meat on a flat pan that allows the juices to run off. There are two ways to remove the salt used to kosher meats. One is to place the raw meat in a large pot filled with cold water and bring the pot to a boil. Then remove the pot from the heat and drain the water. Most of the salt will drain away. Another method is to soak the raw meat, changing the water every 30 minutes.

Your sodium guide

The DASH diet discussed in Chapter 6 outlines the foods and number of servings to eat to reduce your blood pressure. The following guide is meant to complement the DASH diet. It lists foods that are low in sodium and can be eaten more frequently and foods that are high in sodium and should be avoided or eaten only occasionally.

Meat and meat substitutes

Use:

- Fresh or frozen beef, pork, lamb, veal, poultry and wild game without added salt or saline
- Fresh or frozen fish, shrimp, scallops and clams (unbreaded and not packed in brine or with added sodium)

Retraining your taste buds

Your taste for salt is acquired. To unlearn this taste, decrease your use of salt gradually and your taste buds will adjust. Start by using no more than ¼ teaspoon of added salt daily, then gradually decrease to none.

As you use less salt, your preference for it will lessen, allowing you to enjoy the taste of the food itself. Most people find that a few weeks after eliminating salt they no longer miss it.

- Cheese with less than 200 mg sodium per ounce
- Eggs
- No-salt-added peanut butter or unsalted nuts
- No-salt-added canned tuna or other seafood
- Frozen and microwave dinners that have less than 600 mg sodium per dinner

Limit (two or three times a week):

- Regular cottage cheese and mild aged natural cheese, such as brick cheese, Monterey Jack, mild cheddar
- Regular peanut butter
- Canned tuna and other canned seafood packed with 50 percent to 60 percent less salt than usual
- Reduced-sodium processed meats and cheeses
- Lobster and crab

Avoid:

- Meat, fish or poultry that is salt-cured, canned with salt or smoked, such as bacon, chipped beef, corned beef, hot dogs, ham, luncheon meats and sausages
- Processed cheese and cheese spreads
- Pickled herring, eggs and meats
- Salted nuts
- Frozen and microwave dinners that have more than 600 mg sodium per dinner

Fats and oils

Use sparingly:

- Oil, margarine or butter
- Salad dressings with less than 200 mg sodium per serving
- Mayonnaise and unsalted gravy
- Cream cheese, sour cream
- Avocado

Avoid:

- Salad dressings, gravies, spreads and sauces with more than 200 mg of sodium per serving

Milk

Use:

- Milk and yogurt (fat-free or low-fat)

Avoid:

- Commercially cultured buttermilk
- Powdered milk mixes (instant breakfast, cocoa) with more than 200 mg sodium per serving

Grains and starches

Use:

- Grains with less than 200 mg sodium per serving, such as bread, dinner rolls, bagels, English muffins, cereals
- Quick breads such as pancakes or biscuits made from home recipes in which no buttermilk is used and salt is limited or avoided
- Plain muffins
- Crackers with unsalted tops, graham crackers or Melba toast
- Potatoes, rice or pasta
- Unsalted popcorn, pretzels or chips
- Low-sodium canned soups, bouillon and broth

Avoid:

- Grains with more than 200 mg sodium per serving
- Quick breads such as pancakes and biscuits made from commercial mixes
- Salted popcorn, pretzels, chips and crackers
- Regular canned soups, dried soup mixes, broth and bouillon
- Commercially canned and frozen convenience foods (unless labeled low-sodium)
- Commercially prepared refrigerator dough

Vegetables

Use:

- Fresh, unsalted frozen vegetables or no-salt-added canned vegetables
- No-salt-added tomato juice and vegetable juice cocktail
- No-salt-added canned tomato products

About salt substitutes

Before you try a salt substitute, check with your doctor. Some salt substitutes or light salts contain a mixture of sodium chloride (salt) and other compounds. To achieve that familiar salty taste, you may end up using more of the salt substitute than you do regular salt and end up not reducing your sodium intake.

In addition, potassium chloride is a common ingredient in salt substitutes. Too much potassium can be harmful if you have kidney problems or you're taking certain medications to treat high blood pressure or heart failure. Potassium-sparing diuretic drugs cause your kidneys to retain potassium. If you take a potassium-sparing diuretic and use a salt substitute containing potassium, too much potassium can build up in your body. Possible side effects include potentially life-threatening heart rhythm disturbances. Talk with your doctor or a dietitian before using a salt substitute.

Avoid:

- Canned salted tomato products
- Commercially canned and frozen vegetables with added salt
- Salted tomato juice and vegetable juice cocktail
- Sauerkraut and pickled vegetables

Fruits

Use:

- Fresh, frozen and canned fruit

Avoid:

- Fruits dried with a sodium compound

Desserts and sweets

Use:

- Homemade desserts, cooked pudding and box mixes with less than 200 mg sodium per serving
- Fresh fruit, gelatin, fruit ice, sherbet, plain cake, meringue, ice cream and frozen yogurt
- Jams, jellies, honey
- Hard candy, jelly beans

Avoid:

- Box mixes, such as cakes, muffins, cookies, with more than 200 mg sodium per serving
- Desserts and candies prepared with salted nuts
- Refrigerator dough and commercial coffee cakes
- Instant pudding and pie filling mixes, cream or fruit pies

Beverages

Use:

- Bottled water
- Lemonade
- Beverages with less than 70 mg sodium a serving
- Tap water: Sodium content varies with the local water supply.

Chemically softened water may contain added sodium. Discuss use of softened water with a registered dietitian. In most homes, water from the cold tap isn't softened.

Limit (one to two servings per day):

- Coffee and tea
- Cocoa (made with cocoa powder)

Avoid:

- Cocktail beverage mixes, instant beverage mixes such as instant cocoa, commercial sport drinks

Seasonings and condiments

Use:

- Herbs, spices and salt-free herb and spice mixes
- Garlic powder, onion powder and pepper
- Unsalted ketchup, mustard and barbecue sauce
- Lemon juice, flavoring extracts and vinegar
- Prepared horseradish
- Table wine (not cooking wine)

Limit (one or two times a week):

- Regular ketchup or mustard, 1 tablespoon
- Regular bottled meat and barbecue sauces, 1 tablespoon
- Commercial salsa, 1 to 2 tablespoons

Avoid:

- Light-salt products, seasoning salts and mixes, such as celery salt, garlic salt, onion salt
- Meat tenderizer
- Olives and pickles
- Soy sauce, teriyaki sauce and MSG
- Cooking wine

Wrap-up

Key points to remember:

- Sodium significantly increases blood pressure in people who are sensitive to it.
- Approximately 60 percent of people with high blood pressure are sodium sensitive. You're more likely to be sodium sensitive if you're black, age 65 or older, have diabetes or have a family member who is sodium sensitive.
- Whether you have high blood pressure or are healthy, limiting sodium to no more than 2,400 mg daily is reasonable and safe.
- Processed foods generally contain the most sodium. Fresh foods tend to be lower in sodium.
- Instead of salt, use herbs, spices and other flavorings to enhance the flavor of foods.
- Don't use a salt substitute without first talking with your doctor or a dietitian. A salt substitute isn't recommended if you have kidney disease or if you're taking certain medications for high blood pressure or heart failure.

Chapter 6

Eating well

Eating the right kinds of foods can help lower your blood pressure and keep it under control. A healthy diet, along with weight control and physical activity, can lessen the chances you'll need medication to treat your high blood pressure.

Eating well doesn't mean counting calories and giving up all of the foods that you enjoy. It means enjoying a variety of foods that can keep you healthy now and in the years ahead. Eating a variety of foods helps ensure that you get the right mix of nutrients.

To manage high blood pressure, limiting sodium in your diet is important. For more on sodium, see Chapter 5. In addition to limiting sodium, there are other dietary steps to consider. Eating less fat and more grains, fruits, vegetables and low-fat dairy products promotes overall health and has specific blood pressure benefits.

The DASH study

Over the years, several studies have suggested that a healthy diet can reduce your blood pressure. Now there's proof that it's true.

A 1997 study called Dietary Approaches to Stop Hypertension, or DASH, compared three diets among 459 people. The study included people with stage 1 high blood pressure and those with high-normal blood pressure at risk of developing high blood pressure.

Of the three diets in the study, one matched the typical American diet. It was low in fruits, vegetables and dairy products and had a fat content typical of the average American diet (37 percent of total calories). Another diet stressed fruits and vegetables — a minimum of 8 servings — but it didn't control intake of dairy products or fat. The third diet, called the combination diet, stressed fruits and vegetables plus ample grains and low-fat dairy products. Fat also was lower than that of the other diets — less than 30 percent of total calories.

The result was that both the fruit-and-vegetable diet and the combination diet lowered blood pressure. But the combination diet produced the greatest reductions in blood pressure and also lowered total cholesterol.

People with stage 1 high blood pressure on the combination diet experienced an average decrease of 11.4 millimeters of mercury (mm Hg) in systolic pressure and 5.5 mm Hg in diastolic pressure. That's about the same effect as some medications. People with high-normal blood pressure reduced their systolic pressure an average of 3.5 mm Hg and their diastolic pressure an average of 2 mm Hg.

Researchers aren't certain why the combination diet fared better. But they believe it may be because the diet promotes weight loss and because it's rich in potassium, calcium and magnesium, minerals linked with lower blood pressure.

Sodium in all three diets was limited to about 3,000 milligrams (mg) daily — less than what most Americans typically consume. A follow-up study called the DASH-Sodium study found that greater reductions in sodium consumption brought even greater reductions in blood pressure.

Basic principles of DASH

The DASH eating plan is rich in grains, fruits, vegetables and low-fat dairy products. By emphasizing these foods, the plan limits fat, saturated fat and cholesterol while providing plentiful amounts of fiber, potassium, calcium and magnesium. Although research suggests that the DASH diet may specifically help lower high blood pressure, the premise of the diet is similar to Mayo Clinic's Healthy Weight Pyramid (see page 91), which is designed to help you manage your weight. Both plans promote eating more grains, which contain fiber and complex carbohydrates, more fruits and vegetables, and fewer animal products, including meat, poultry and fish.

The DASH plan differs in that it separates vegetable proteins from animal proteins, recommending four to five servings a week of nuts, seeds and legumes. In this way, the DASH diet helps ensure more fiber, plus potassium and magnesium, nutrients associated with lower blood pressure.

How to eat with DASH

To manage your blood pressure with your diet, here are the types and amounts of foods to eat every day:

Grains: 7 to 8 servings. Grains include breads, cereals, rice and pasta. Whole grains provide more fiber and nutrients, such as magnesium, than refined varieties provide. In addition to being low in fat, grains are rich in complex carbohydrates and nutrients.

Breads and pasta are naturally low in fat and calories. To keep them that way, be selective about what you add to these foods. Avoid cream and cheese sauces on pasta and choose instead vegetable or fresh tomato-based sauces. Select plain yeast breads rather than quick breads, sweet rolls or other baked goods with added fat.

Fruits and vegetables: 8 to 10 servings. Eating more fruits and vegetables may be one of the best things you can do to improve your blood pressure and your overall health. In addition to being virtually fat-free and low in calories, fruits and vegetables provide fiber and a variety of nutrients, including potassium and magnesium. They also contain phytochemicals, substances that may help reduce your risk of cardiovascular disease and some cancers.

Substituting fruits and vegetables for foods that have more fat and calories is also a relatively easy way to improve your diet without cutting back on the amount you eat. The key is not to smother your fruits and vegetables with dips or sauces that contain a lot of fat.

Dairy products: 2 to 3 servings. Dairy products are key sources of calcium and vitamin D, which help your body absorb calcium.

The DASH diet

This is the plan that reduced blood pressure by the greatest amount in the DASH study. To help control your blood pressure, try to eat daily the amounts listed from the different food groups.

Food & daily servings	Serving examples
Grains 7 to 8	½ cup (3 oz/90 g) cooked cereal, rice or pasta ½ cup (1 oz/30 g) ready-to-eat cereal 1 slice whole-wheat (wholemeal) sandwich bread ½ bagel or English muffin
Fruits & vegetables 8 to 10	¼ cup (1½ oz/45 g) raisins ¾ cup (6 fl oz/180 mL) 100 percent fruit juice 1 medium apple or banana 12 grapes 1 cup (2 oz/60 g) raw leafy green vegetables ½ cup (3 oz/90 g) cooked vegetables 1 medium potato
Dairy products 2 to 3	1 cup (8 fl oz/250 mL) low-fat or fat-free milk or 1 cup (8 oz/250 g) yogurt 1½ oz (45 g) reduced-fat or fat-free cheese 2 cups (16 oz/500 g) low-fat or fat-free cottage cheese
Meat, poultry & fish 2 or fewer	2 to 3 oz (60 to 90 g) cooked skinless poultry, seafood or lean meat
Legumes, nuts & seeds 4 to 5 a week	½ cup (3 ½ oz/105 g) cooked legumes ¼ cup (1 oz/30 g) seeds ⅓ cup (1 oz/30 g) nuts

Because it's not always convenient to measure your food, here are some tips to help you eat the right portions:

1 cup = the size of your fist
3 oz = the size of a deck of cards
1 oz = 1 to 2 handfuls
1 tsp = the tip of your thumb
1 tbsp = 3 thumb tips

Serving amounts are based on a diet of 2,000 calories a day. Most Americans need between 1,600 and 2,400 calories daily, depending on age and activity. To adjust the diet to include fewer or more servings, talk to a registered dietitian.

The DASH diet may be found on the National Heart, Lung, and Blood Institute Web site at *www.nhlbi.nih.gov*. Search the term "DASH diet."

Adapted from the National Institutes of Health, *The DASH Diet*, 2001.

They also provide protein. But dairy products can be high in fat. By choosing low-fat or fat-free varieties, such as skim or low-fat milk and yogurt, and fat-free or part-skim cheeses, you can get the health benefits of dairy products without all the fat. *Note:* If you are lactose intolerant and have difficulty digesting dairy foods, you may benefit from products containing the enzyme lactase, which can reduce or prevent the symptoms of lactose intolerance.

Meat, poultry and fish: 2 or fewer servings (6 ounces or less daily). These foods are rich sources of protein, B vitamins, magnesium, iron and zinc. When you do eat meat, choose lean cuts, such as tenderloin, round or sirloin. When preparing poultry, remove the skin to reduce fat by about half. However, because even lean varieties contain fat and cholesterol, try to limit all animal foods. Fish is one of the healthiest animal proteins you can choose. Some fish contain high amounts of omega-3 fatty acids, which have been shown to reduce the risk of sudden death by lowering the risk of

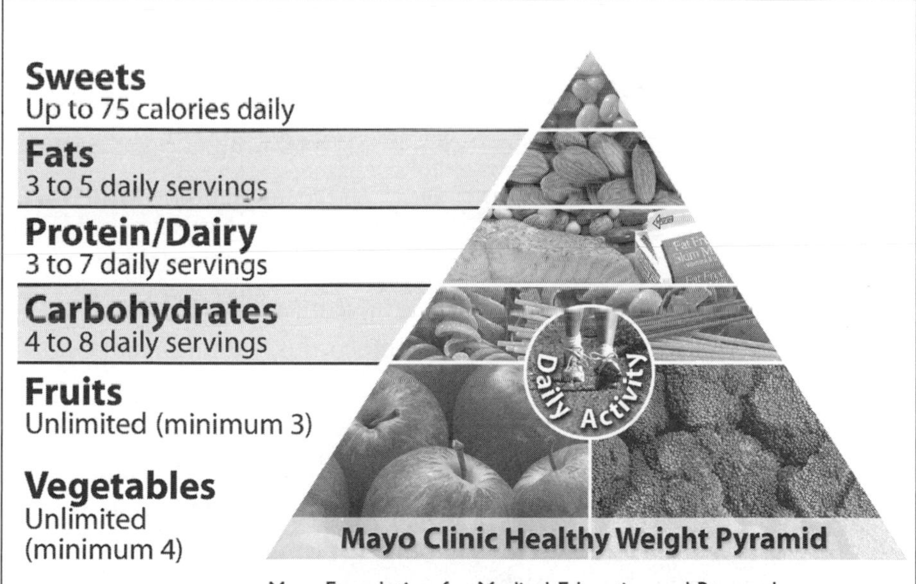

The DASH diet is similar in many respects to Mayo Clinic's Healthy Weight Pyramid — the principles of which provide a healthy eating plan for most Americans. Both emphasize greater consumption of fruits, vegetables and carbohydrate-containing grains and less consumption of meat.

abnormal heart rhythms. For other benefits of omega-3 fatty acids, see "Get the skinny on fatty acids" on page 100.

Legumes, nuts and seeds: 4 to 5 servings a week. Legumes include beans, dried peas and lentils, which are low in fat and have no cholesterol. They're an excellent source of plant protein. Legumes, nuts and seeds provide a variety of nutrients, including magnesium and potassium, plus phytochemicals and fiber.

Although nuts and seeds contain fat, most of it is monounsaturated, the type that may help protect against coronary artery disease.

Menus with DASH

To help you get started on a healthier diet, see the menus and recipes in the back of this book that incorporate the DASH eating plan. They begin on page 191.

Three important minerals

The DASH diet emphasizes the benefits of three minerals — potassium, calcium and magnesium — that are key factors in managing high blood pressure. This table summarizes the effects of the minerals on blood pressure and what foods contain them.

Mineral	How it works	Where it's found
Potassium	Balances the amount of sodium in your cells.	Many fruits and vegetables, whole grains, legumes, dairy products.
Calcium	Not proved to prevent high blood pressure, but eating too little is linked with high blood pressure.	Dairy products, green leafy vegetables, fish with edible bones, calcium-fortified foods.
Magnesium	A deficiency is linked with higher blood pressure.	Legumes, green leafy vegetables, nuts and seeds, whole grains, lean meats.

Good sources of potassium

These foods have moderate to very high amounts of potassium in each serving. You'll find that some foods are listed more than once, due to how they're prepared or preserved.

	Fruits	Vegetables	Other
Moderate	Apple, raw	Asparagus (6 spears)	
	Blackberries	Broccoflower	
	Cherries, sour, canned	Broccoli	
	Grapefruit	Cabbage	
	Grapes	Carrots, canned or raw	
	Mandarin orange	Corn	
	Peaches, canned or fresh	Eggplant	
	Pear, fresh	Green beans	
	Pineapple, canned or fresh	Kale	
	Plums, canned or fresh	Lettuce	
	Raisins (2 tbsp)	Mixed vegetables, frozen	
	Strawberries	Peas, fresh or frozen	
		Rhubarb, fresh or frozen	
		Turnips	
		Squash (summer)	
		Sweet potato	
High	Apple juice	Artichoke	Cocoa mixes, ¼ cup (1 oz/30 g) powder
	Apricot nectar	Bamboo shoots	Milk, 1 cup (8 fl oz/250 mL)
	Apricots, whole (4) and dried	Beans, dried	Peanut butter, (2 tbsp)
	Banana (½)	Beets	Tofu (½ cup)
	Cantaloupe	Broccoli	Yogurt, 1 cup (8 oz/250 g)
	Cherries, sweet red	Brussels sprouts	
	Dates (4)	Collard greens cooked	
	Elderberries	Kohlrabi, cooked	
	Figs, raw, dried (2)	Mixed vegetables, canned	
	Grapefruit juice		

Good sources of potassium (continued)

	Fruits	Vegetables	Other
	Grape juice	Mushrooms	
	Guava	Okra	
	Honeydew	Parsley	
	Kiwi	Parsnips, cooked	
	Mango	Potato, cooked, mashed or plain chips	
	Nectarine	Pumpkin	
	Orange	Rutabaga, cooked	
	Orange juice	Spinach	
	Papaya	Squash	
	Pineapple juice	Sweet potato, canned	
	Prunes	Tomato, canned whole or spaghetti sauce	
	Tangerines (2)	Vegetable juice cocktail	
		Wax beans, canned	
		Zucchini	
Very high	Passion fruit juice	Avocado	Chocolate milk, 1 cup (8 fl oz/ 250 mL)
	Prune Juice	Bamboo shoots, raw	Potassium chloride salt substitutes, 1⁄4 tsp
	Tomato juice	Carrot juice	
		Chicory	
		Potato, baked	
		Sweet potato, baked	
		Swiss chard, boiled	
		Water chestnuts	

Your 15 best sources of calcium

It's recommended that most adults get between 1,000 mg and 1,500 mg of calcium daily. Here are some of the foods that can help you reach that amount.

	Calcium (milligrams)
Milk, fat-free and low-fat, 1 cup (8 fl oz/250 mL)	300
Tofu set with calcium, 1/2 cup (4 oz/125 g) — check label	200 to 800
Yogurt, 1 cup (8 oz/250 g)	350
Orange juice, calcium-fortified, 1 cup (8 fl oz/250 mL)	300
Ready-to-eat cereal, calcium-fortified, 1 cup (1 1/2 oz/45 g)	200
Mozzarella cheese, part-skim, 1/4 cup (1 oz/30 g)	183
Canned salmon with bones (3 oz/90 g)	203
Collard greens, cooked, 1/2 cup (3 oz/90 g)	113
Ricotta cheese, part-skim, 1/4 cup (2 oz/60 g)	169
Bread, calcium-fortified, 2 slices	160
Cottage cheese, low-fat, 1 cup (8 oz/250 g)	150
Parmesan cheese, 2 tbsp	138
Navy beans, cooked, 1 cup (7 oz/220 g)	128
Turnip greens, cooked, 1 cup (3 oz/90 g)	197
Broccoli, cooked, 1 cup (2 oz/60 g)	94

What about supplements?

A healthy diet should provide adequate potassium, calcium and magnesium. Studies have shown that getting these nutrients from foods instead of supplements helps ensure the right mix of the nutrients that only food can provide.

If you're taking a diuretic (di-u-RET-ik) medication that causes your body to lose potassium, your doctor may recommend a potassium supplement if your diet isn't providing enough. Note that over-the-counter potassium supplements can have serious side effects, such as digestive tract laceration. In addition, some classes of antihypertensive medications, such as potassium-retaining diuretcs, angiotensin converting enzyme inhibitors and angiotensin receptor blockers, can increase potassium in your blood. Take potassium supplements only if your doctor recommends them.

Calcium and magnesium supplements generally aren't necessary to control high blood pressure. If you have kidney disease, ask your doctor about minerals in your diet.

Common sources of magnesium

Magnesium is found in a wide variety of foods and in drinking water. Regularly eating green leafy vegetables, whole grains, legumes and even small amounts of meat, poultry and fish will ensure you get an adequate amount. Nuts and seeds also are good sources of magnesium.

A fresh approach to shopping

When you go grocery shopping, think fresh and unprocessed. Try to spend most of your time shopping the perimeter of the store where fresh produce, dairy and meat items are located. Here are some tips to help you follow the DASH eating plan:

Plan. Decide on the meals you're going to make during the coming week and include the ingredients you need on your grocery list. Don't forget about what you'll need for breakfast and snacks. Plan to include more fruits, vegetables, whole-grain breads and cereals on your list. Occasionally, try legumes such as lentils, kidney or lima beans as your source of protein.

Buy fresh. Fresh foods are generally better than ready-to-eat foods because you can control what ingredients are added. In addition, fresh foods generally have more flavor and color and less sodium.

Don't shop on an empty stomach. If you shop when you're hungry, you may be tempted to buy foods you don't need, and these may be high in fat, calories and sodium.

Read the labels. Take time to read food labels. They can help you compare similar foods and select items that are the most nutritious.

How to use food labels

Since May 1994, packaged goods sold in the United States have carried the Nutrition Facts label. Nutrition Facts are an at-a-glance method for verifying how a food fits into your eating plan.

Each label contains information pertaining to:

Serving size. Look at the serving size and servings per container. See if the serving size is similar to the amount you actually eat. If you eat more, then the amount of calories and nutrients you get from that item will be higher. If you eat less, the amount will be lower.

Calories from fat. Use this information to compare products and to add up the amount of fat you eat. Limit fat to about 65 grams a day. This amount keeps fat at the recommended level — less than 30 percent of your daily calories, based on a 2,000-calorie diet.

Nutrition Facts sample label

Serving size ½ cup (114 g)
Servings per container 4

Amount per serving	
Calories 90	Calories from fat 30
	Percent Daily Value*
Total fat 3 g	5%
Saturated fat 0 g	0%
Cholesterol 0 mg	0%
Sodium 300 mg	13%
Total carbohydrate 13 g	4%
Dietary fiber 3 g	12%
Sugars 3 g	
Protein 3 g	

Vitamin A	80%	Vitamin C	60%
Calcium	4%	Iron	4%

*Percent Daily Values are based on a 2,000-calorie diet. Your daily values may be higher or lower depending on your calorie needs:

	Calories	2,000	2,500
Total fat	Less than	65 g	80 g
Saturated fat	Less than	20 g	25 g
Cholesterol	Less than	300 mg	300 mg
Sodium	Less than	2,400 mg	2,400 mg
Total carbohydrate		300 g	375 g
Fiber		25 g	30 g

Calories per gram:
Fat 9 Carbohydrates 4 Protein 4

Daily value. These values represent the amounts of nutrients and fiber desirable in 2,000- and 2,500-calorie diets. The Percent Daily Value tells you how much of the recommended daily amount 1 serving contains, based on 2,000 calories.

For fat, saturated fat and cholesterol, choose foods with a low-percent daily value. For total carbohydrate, dietary fiber, vitamins and minerals, try to reach 100 percent of the daily value of each.

Sodium. Because as much as 90 percent of the sodium that Americans consume comes from processed foods, it's important to chose foods with less than 200 mg of sodium a serving, or under 8 percent daily value serving.

Stocking your kitchen

You're more likely to prepare healthy dishes if you have everything you need in your kitchen. You don't need unusual or hard-to-find ingredients to eat well. You're likely to find everything you need at a well-stocked supermarket.

Here are examples of good foods to keep on hand:

Dairy products
Low-fat or fat-free milk
Low-fat or fat-free cottage cheese or ricotta
Reduced-fat cheeses
Reduced-fat or fat-free sour cream
Tub or squeeze margarine

Grains
Whole-grain bread, bagels, pita bread
Low-fat flour tortillas
Plain, whole-grain cereal, dry or cooked
Rice, brown or white
Pasta, noodles and spaghetti
Whole-grain crackers

Fruits
Standard fresh varieties
Seasonal fresh fruits
Canned fruit in juice or water
Frozen fruit without added sugar
Dried fruit

Vegetables
Standard fresh varieties
Seasonal fresh vegetables
Frozen vegetables without added butter or sauces
Canned tomato products low in sodium
Canned vegetables or vegetable soups low in sodium

Legumes (without added salt)
Lentils
Black beans
Red (kidney) beans
Navy beans
Chickpeas (garbanzos)

Meat
White meat, skinless chicken and turkey
Fish (unbreaded)
Pork tenderloin
Extra-lean ground beef
Round or sirloin beef cuts

Baking items
Imitation butter, flakes or buds
Nonstick cooking spray
Canned evaporated milk, fat-free or reduced-fat
Cocoa powder, unsweetened
Angel food cake mix

Condiments, seasonings and spreads
Low-fat or fat-free salad dressings (choose those lowest in sodium)
Herbs
Spices
Flavored vinegars
Salsa or picante sauce

Healthy cooking techniques

Once you have your kitchen stocked with fresh, healthy foods, cooking becomes easy and fun. Begin by broiling or grilling meat or fish seasoned with herbs. Bake a potato and add a fresh green salad with tomato and green pepper. Have a glass of skim milk and some fresh fruit for dessert, and you've created a low-fat, low-sodium meal that's highly nutritious.

To manage high blood pressure and improve your health, try to cook without salt and little or no oils or other fats.

Here are some tips to get you started:

- Use unsoftened water for drinking and cooking.
- To enhance a food's flavor without adding salt or fat, use fresh onions, herbs, spices, peppers, garlic, ginger, lemons and limes, flavored vinegars, and reduced-sodium soy sauce.
- Dress up vegetables with herbs, spices or butter-flavored powders, instead of salt or butter.
- Cut the amount of meat in stews and casseroles by a third and add more vegetables, rice or pasta.
- In recipes, substitute lower-fat dairy products, such as reduced-fat cream cheese and sour cream, for their higher-fat counterparts.

- To replace all or part of the sugar in recipes, use cinnamon, nutmeg, vanilla and fruit. They enhance sweetness.
- Invest in nonstick cookware to saute or brown foods without adding fat. If you normally add a tablespoon of vegetable oil to a skillet, you can save 120 calories and 14 grams of fat by using a nonstick skillet instead. Or use a vegetable oil cooking spray. It only adds about 1 gram of fat and few calories.
- Saute onions, mushrooms or celery in a small amount of low-sodium broth or water instead of butter or oil.
- Grill, broil, poach, roast or stir-fry your foods instead of frying them.
- Cook fish in parchment paper or foil. This seals in flavor and juices.

Get the skinny on fatty acids

Most plans for healthy eating call on you to sharply limit the amount of saturated fat you consume. However, you may hear about other kinds of fats — in particular, trans-fatty acids and omega-3 fatty acids. Knowing the difference between them can help you meet your goals for treating high blood pressure.

Trans-fatty acids. Because they can increase the risk of cardiovascular disease, this is one class of fats to avoid. Trans-fatty acids are found in partially hydrogenated oils. Look for these oils as ingredients in crackers, cookies and fast foods. Checking food labels can help you steer clear of these bad fats.

Omega-3 fatty acids. Some fish — particularly fatty types prevalent in cold water, such as salmon, mackerel and herring — contain high amounts of omega-3 fatty acids. Omega-3s are also present in smaller amounts in green leafy vegetables, soybeans, nuts, flaxseed and canola oil.

Omega-3 fatty acids offer a good form of fat. They may:

- Lower your blood triglyceride level. If your triglyceride level is extremely high and doesn't respond to prescribed medication, your doctor may suggest that you use a fish oil supplement in addition to your medication. This is the only use of fish oil capsules supported by the American Heart Association.

- Reduce your risk of blood clots. Omega-3 fatty acids act as a natural anticoagulant by altering the ability of platelets in your blood to clump together. The platelets become less sticky, so clot formation is less likely. Blood clots that form in narrowed arteries increase your risk of a heart attack or stroke.
- Lower blood pressure. Several studies have examined the effects of omega-3 fatty acids on blood pressure. Those who eat fish tend to have a lower incidence of borderline or high blood pressure.

Dietitians generally recommend at least two meals of fish every week for possible heart benefits.

Fish oil capsules aren't a good substitute for fish. In high doses they pose risks, especially if you're regularly taking aspirin or a blood thinner, such as warfarin (Coumadin, Panwarfin). Before you take fish oil capsules, consult with your doctor.

It's important for women who are or who can become pregnant to know that some fish contain high levels of methylmercury. Regularly eating this form of mercury can harm a fetus' developing nervous system. To avoid this danger, the Food and Drug Administration offers these guidelines:

- Don't eat large fish that can contain high levels of methylmercury. These include shark, swordfish, king mackerel and tilefish.
- Eat a variety of fish — shellfish, canned fish, smaller ocean fish or farm-raised fish. You can safely eat 12 ounces a week of cooked fish. A typical serving size of fish is from 3 to 6 ounces.
- Check with your state or local health department for special advisories on fish caught from waters in your local area.

Eating well when eating out

You can eat nutritiously away from home too. The most important thing is to continue with the healthy choices that you've begun in planning menus at home. Remember that eating out isn't a time to forget all you know about choosing healthy foods. In fact, dining out can be a great opportunity to try new foods.

Many restaurants provide healthy food choices. Some restaurants even reserve a special section of their menu for healthier fare. Many restaurants will honor special requests to prepare an item with less fat and sodium.

If the entree is larger than you want, ask if you can have the lunch portion, even if you're eating dinner. You can also request a take-home bag when the meal is served. That way you can reserve half the meal for the next day. Or you might choose an appetizer for an entree or split a meal with a companion.

What to order

Following these suggestions will help you keep your eating plan on target when you're away from home:

Appetizer. Choose appetizers with vegetables, fruit or fish, such as chopped, raw vegetables, fresh-fruit compote or shrimp cocktail (use lemon juice instead of cocktail sauce).

Soup. You're often better off avoiding soup and choosing fruit or a salad. Broth or tomato-based soups are often high in sodium. Creamed soups, chowders, pureed soups and some fruit soups contain heavy cream and egg yolks.

Salad. Order lettuce or spinach salads with dressings on the side and limit yourself to one soup spoon of dressing. Caesar salads are high in fat, cholesterol and sodium. Chef salads also are high in fat, cholesterol and calories because of the amount of cheese, eggs and meat they contain. Taco salads typically aren't a good choice because they contain high-fat items such as cheese, guacamole, ground beef and a fried shell.

Bread. If you're offered a bread basket, choose whole-grain bread, rolls, breadsticks or bagels. Eat them plain or with a little honey, jam or jelly. These fat-free toppings contribute few calories

Check out MayoClinic.com for healthy recipes

Visit our Web site at *www.MayoClinic.com* to browse through recipes for great-tasting dishes that are low in fat and sodium and rich in nutrients. You can find the recipes in the Food & Nutrition Center.

when used sparingly. Muffins, garlic toast or croissants have more fat. Crackers can be high in sodium and fat.

Entree. Look for entrees with descriptions that indicate low-fat content, such as London broil, grilled chicken breast, lemon-baked fish or broiled beef kabobs.

Avoid items with descriptions indicating higher-fat content, such as prime rib of beef, veal parmigiana, stuffed shrimp, fried chicken or filet mignon with bearnaise sauce, creamed vegetables and cream sauces. If you're not sure how much fat is in the sauce you're ordering, ask for it on the side so that you can control how much you add.

Side dish. Choose a baked potato, boiled new potatoes, steamed vegetables, rice or fresh fruit instead of french fries, potato chips, onion rings or mayonnaise-based salads, such as potato salad. Ask that no butter, margarine or salt be used to prepare the vegetable or rice.

Condiments. Choose items like fresh tomato, cucumber and lettuce for your sandwiches. Avoid olives, pickles and sauerkraut because of their high-sodium content. Use ketchup, mustard and mayonnaise sparingly.

Dessert. Choose fresh fruit, poached spiced fruit, plain cake with fruit puree, or sorbet or sherbet.

Alcohol. Alcohol is high in fat and calories. Excessive alcohol can also increase your blood pressure. If you choose to drink alcohol, limit the amount to one drink a day if you're a woman and one or two drinks if you're a man. Alcohol's relationship to high blood pressure is discussed further in Chapter 8.

Putting it in perspective

If all of the suggestions in this chapter seem a bit overwhelming, remember that eating well isn't an all-or-nothing proposition. Each food you eat doesn't have to be perfect. Perfection isn't the goal — being persistent in your pursuit of healthy eating is what's important. Over time, this approach to eating well will become a habit that will help you manage your high blood pressure and feel better too.

Wrap-up

Key points to remember:

- A healthy diet can reduce your blood pressure as much as some medications.
- The DASH diet can help lower blood pressure by promoting generous amounts of whole grains, fruits, vegetables and low-fat dairy products. The diet is low in sodium and fat and high in potassium, calcium and magnesium — nutrients associated with lower blood pressure.
- It's easier to eat well when you plan your meals, read food labels and stock up on nutritious ingredients.
- When cooking, use little or no salt, fats or oils. Instead, use herbs and spices to enhance the flavor of your food.
- When eating out, look for dishes low in fat and sodium and ask for what you want.

Chapter 7

Getting more active

One of the most important things you can do to reduce your blood pressure is to become more physically active. Regular activity can lower your blood pressure by about the same amount as many blood pressure medications.

A major reason high blood pressure is so common is that people aren't active enough. Modern conveniences and a shortage of free time have caused Americans to become increasingly sedentary. According to the American Heart Association, only 27 percent of Americans age 18 and older get enough exercise to help their cardiovascular fitness. About 44 percent get some exercise, but not enough for heart benefits. And about 28 percent get no leisure-time physical activity at all.

To lower your blood pressure, you don't have to become an athlete. The motto of physical fitness used to be "No pain, no gain." But no more. Moderate activities also can be beneficial to your blood pressure and overall health, provided you do them regularly. What's important is including more physical activity in your daily routine, not great exhibits of endurance.

Physical activity and blood pressure

Physical activity is critical to controlling your blood pressure because it makes your heart stronger. Your heart is able to pump more blood with less effort. And the less your heart has to work to pump blood, the less force that's exerted on your arteries. In addition, regular activity also helps promote weight loss.

Regular physical activity can lower your blood pressure by 5 to 10 millimeters of mercury (mm Hg). If you're at risk of high blood pressure, that's enough to keep the condition from developing. If you have high blood pressure, it may be enough to prevent you from having to take medication. If you're taking medication, it's enough to make your medication work more effectively.

In addition to helping control your blood pressure, regular activity also reduces your risk of heart attack, high cholesterol, diabetes, osteoporosis and some cancers.

Your blood pressure may stay at a temporarily low level for some time after exercising. To get a true picture of where it's at, remember that if you're doing home monitoring, measure your blood pressure before you exercise instead of afterward.

Activity vs. intensity

For many years, the common belief was that you had to exercise vigorously if you wanted to become physically fit and improve your health. As a result, people developed an all-or-nothing attitude toward exercise. But studies show that even light activity is good for your blood pressure and overall health — and it's definitely better than doing nothing at all.

In 2002, the Department of Health and Human Services issued guidelines urging Americans to take part in regular physical activity. *Activity* is often the preferred term to *exercise* because to many people, exercise implies a planned and repetitive routine. An activity doesn't have to be structured to be beneficial.

These federal guidelines recommend a minimum of one of the following:

- 30 to 60 minutes of moderate activity on at least 5 days a week

- 20 minutes of vigorous physical activity at least three times a week.

In addition to common forms of physical activity, such as walking or bicycling, the new guidelines promote activities such as mowing your lawn with a push mower, scrubbing floors or going dancing. You can also accumulate your activities throughout the day. Ride your bike to the convenience store or spend a few minutes working in your flower bed.

However, not all daily activities count. The activity should be moderately intense. That equates to an effort you perceive as being fairly light to somewhat hard.

The change in emphasis from exercise to activity doesn't discount the benefits of vigorous exercise. The new guidelines are meant to complement — not replace — previous advice promoting high-intensity activities. More-strenuous activity brings even greater health benefits. The main point is that you take part in some type of physical activity for 30 to 60 minutes most days of the week.

Perceived exertion scale

Moderately intense physical activity qualifies as fairly light to somewhat hard, or about 11 to 14, on the perceived exertion scale. Perceived exertion refers to the total amount of effort, physical stress and fatigue you perceive during an activity.

6	
7	Very, very light
8	
9	Very light
10	
11	Fairly light
12	
13	Somewhat hard
14	
15	Hard
16	
17	Very hard
18	
19	Very, very hard
20	

What kind of activity?

Total fitness involves three components — aerobic activity to improve your heart and lung capacity (cardiovascular health), flexibility exercises to improve flexibility in your joints, and strengthening exercises to maintain bone and muscle mass.

Of these three, aerobic activity has the greatest effect on controlling your blood pressure. An activity is aerobic if it places added demands on your heart, lungs and muscles, increasing your need for oxygen.

Cleaning house, playing golf or raking leaves all are aerobic activities if they require a fairly light to somewhat hard effort. Other common forms of aerobic activity include:

Walking. Walking is appealing to many people because it doesn't require any special athletic skills or instruction. It's convenient and inexpensive. You can vary your route to keep it interesting. And it's an activity that you can enjoy alone or with friends.

Walking also helps burn calories. You burn about an equal amount of fat during long-duration, low-intensity exercise as you do during short exercise periods.

When walking, make sure you wear good shoes that give your feet support and traction. If you've been inactive and are out of shape, begin by walking at a very light pace (see "Perceived exertion scale") for 5 to 10 minutes. Each time you walk, gradually increase the intensity and duration, as you can tolerate it.

Jogging. Jogging is an excellent form of aerobic exercise because it works your heart, lungs and muscles in a relatively brief time. This allows many people to fit jogging into their busy schedules. And, like walking, jogging doesn't require a lot of equipment — just a good pair of shoes.

However, jogging requires prior cardiovascular conditioning and muscle strengthening. If you have arthritis, it can contribute to pain or discomfort in your knees, hips or ankles.

If you'd like to start jogging but you haven't been active for several months, begin by walking. When you're able to walk 2 miles (1.6 kilometers) in 30 minutes comfortably, you're ready to try alternating jogging with walking. Gradually increase the amount of time you spend jogging and decrease the amount of time you spend walking. To minimize your risk of injury and muscle and joint discomfort, don't jog more than three or four times a week and try to jog on alternate days.

Bicycling. Like walking, bicycling is a good choice if you're just getting started on a regular exercise program. Start slowly and build up your endurance. You may be tempted to challenge yourself by setting the gears to make pedaling hard, producing a strain resembling that of a hard run. This doesn't work your heart and lungs effectively, except when you're ascending a hill. Pedaling more rapidly at all times — 80 to 100 revolutions per minute — will help make your ride more aerobic.

Swimming. Swimming is an excellent form of cardiovascular exercise because it conditions your heart, lungs and muscles throughout your body. It's also gentle to your joints. If you have arthritis or another joint disease, swimming is a good way to increase your aerobic activity.

Exercise machines. There are a variety of exercise machines to help you build aerobic capacity. In general, you get what you pay for when you purchase an exercise machine. Look at the warranty — it's usually a sign of quality. Make sure the device is solidly built, with no exposed cables or chains. Avoid spring-operated components, and look for a machine that operates smoothly.

Each of these six basic machines offers unique fitness benefits:

Stationary bicycle. This is an excellent choice for both beginning and veteran exercisers. It gives you mainly a lower-body workout, but some bicycles have moving handlebars that also provide an upper-body workout, increasing demands on your heart and lungs. If you have knee problems, be sure the resistance can be adjusted to a low setting, and keep your knees bent throughout the pedaling cycle.

Rowing machine. This machine offers a good aerobic workout by exercising muscles throughout your body, as well as your heart and lungs. It exercises your back, shoulders, stomach, legs and arms. Machines with a flywheel and chain drive generally are easier to operate and are more effective than piston-type rowers, which are less expensive and more compact. Proper technique is important to avoid back strain.

Treadmill. A treadmill lets you walk, jog or run indoors. Some models offer adjustable inclines that simulate climbing hills. You can adjust the speed for walking or jogging. High horsepower models generally run smoother and are more durable.

Stair climber. This helps exercise your hips, buttocks, thighs, hamstrings, calves and lower back. A stair climber also provides an effective heart and lung workout. Compared with jogging, it reduces wear and tear on your ankles and knees. Still, the device can aggravate existing knee problems.

Cross-country ski machine. Advantages of this machine are that it offers a good overall workout and it's easy on your joints. But some people find it difficult to master. You have to be able to move your arms and legs in rhythmic opposition. This can take practice.

Elliptical machine. The low-impact movements of an elliptical offer a good aerobic workout while building leg strength. The elliptical motion minimizes impact to your hips, knees, feet and lower back while exercising the muscles of your lower body.

How much activity?

Be as active as you can each day. At a minimum, aim to burn at least 150 calories daily doing aerobic activities. For moderately intense activities, that equals about 30 minutes. Lighter activities require more time, and more vigorous activities less time. In addition, the more you weigh, the less time it takes to burn calories — the less you weigh, the more time. However, if you use 30 minutes as your guide, you'll be close to getting the minimal amount of activity you need. (See "Activity guide" on page 111.)

If it's difficult to carve 30 minutes out of your busy schedule, you can accumulate your activities in 5- to 10-minute intervals throughout the day. Park your car farther away from work. Take the stairs instead of the elevator. Go for a short walk during your lunch hour and schedule walking meetings with a colleague or two. Three 10-minute periods of activity are almost as beneficial to your overall fitness as one 30-minute session.

In addition, look for opportunities to include more activity within your regular routine. While watching or listening to the news, walk on your treadmill. When reading a magazine or book, get on your stationary bicycle.

The six-step fitness plan below outlines how to start an activity program, how to add time or distance as your fitness improves and how to add strength training to round out your overall fitness.

Activity guide

Activity	Minutes required to burn 150 calories in 155-pound person*
Washing and waxing a car	45 to 60
Washing windows and floors	45 to 60
Playing volleyball	45
Playing touch football	30 to 45
Gardening	30 to 45
Wheeling self in wheelchair	30 to 40
Walking (20 minutes per mile)	35
Basketball (shooting baskets)	30
Bicycling (6 minutes per mile)	30
Dancing fast	30
Raking leaves	30
Water aerobics	30
Lawn mowing (push mower)	30
Walking (15 minutes per mile)	30
Swimming laps	20
Basketball (playing a game)	15 to 20
Jogging (12 minutes per mile)	20
Running (10 minutes per mile)	15
Shoveling snow	15
Stair climbing	15

*Equivalent to minutes required to burn 630 calories in 154 pound person. Adapted from National Institutes of Health. *Clinical Guidelines on the Identification, Evaluation, and Treatment of Overweight and Obesity in Adults,* 1998.

A 6-step fitness plan

One of the challenges of incorporating more physical activity into your day is just getting out of your chair and doing it. You know that you should be more active, but taking that first step to being more active sometimes isn't as easy as it may seem.

To help you get and stay active, here's a fitness program that's safe for most people. However, if you have any chronic health conditions or you're at significant risk of cardiovascular disease, some special precautions may apply. To be on the safe side, check with your doctor first if you:

- Have a blood pressure of 160/100 mm Hg or more
- Have cardiovascular or lung disease, diabetes, arthritis, osteoporosis or kidney disease
- Are a man age 40 years or older or a woman age 50 or older
- Have a family history of heart-related problems before age 55
- Are unsure of your health status
- Have previously experienced chest discomfort, shortness of breath or dizziness during times when you've exerted yourself

If you take medication regularly, ask your doctor if increasing your physical activity will change how the medication works or its side effects. Drugs for diabetes and cardiovascular disease can sometimes cause dehydration, impaired balance and blurred vision. Some medications can also affect the way your body reacts to exercise.

Step 1: Set your goals

Goals help motivate you to get and stay active. Start with simple goals, such as trying to be active most days of the week, and then progress to longer-range goals. People who can stay physically active for 6 months usually end up making regular activity a habit.

Be sure to set goals you can reasonably achieve. It's easy to get frustrated and give up on goals that are too ambitious. Plus, be specific about your goals. State exactly what your goal is and the time you want to achieve it.

If you have, or are at risk of, high blood pressure, one of your goals should be to lower your blood pressure. Another goal might be to lose weight. Your goals might read as follows:

- I will lower my systolic blood pressure by 4 mm Hg and my diastolic pressure by 2 mm Hg in 6 months.
- I will lose 5 pounds (2.7 kilograms) in 6 months.

To achieve these health goals, it may help you to set some activity goals. These goals should also be attainable and specific. Here are some examples:

- I will stretch before and after physical activity.
- I will walk for 30 to 60 minutes 3 days a week.
- I will do strengthening exercises 2 days a week.

Once you've decided on your goals, write them down and keep them where you can see them. Seeing your goals can help motivate you. As you accomplish your goals, set new ones.

Step 2: Assemble your equipment

Your equipment can be as simple as athletic shoes. Wear shoes that fit your feet well and provide good support.

If you plan to bicycle, make sure your bicycle is adjusted for your height and arm length. When you are seated and have your foot on the pedal nearest the ground, your leg should be not quite fully extended. You should also be able to reach the handlebars and work the brakes and shift mechanism while keeping your eyes on the road.

If you decide to purchase an exercise machine, learn how to adjust it to fit your size and level of endurance.

For strength training, you can make your own weights by filling old socks with beans or pennies, or partially filling a half-gallon milk jug with water or sand. Or you can purchase used weights by the pound at some athletic equipment stores. A resistance band can help you work major muscle groups.

Step 3: Take time to stretch

Stretching for 5 to 10 minutes before you begin an activity increases blood flow and limbers up your muscles. This helps prepare your body for your upcoming aerobic activity. Be sure to warm up briefly before you stretch because stretching a cold muscle can strain and irritate tissue.

Stretching for 5 to 10 minutes after an aerobic activity — when your muscles are loosened up — improves flexibility in muscles and joints. It also helps prevent muscle soreness and reduces risk of injury.

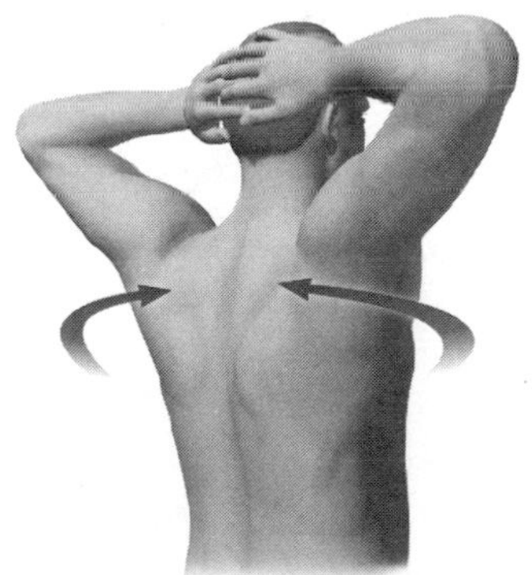

Chest stretch: Clasp your hands behind your head. Pull elbows firmly back while inhaling deeply. Hold for 30 seconds (keep breathing). Relax.

More warm-up and cool-down stretches

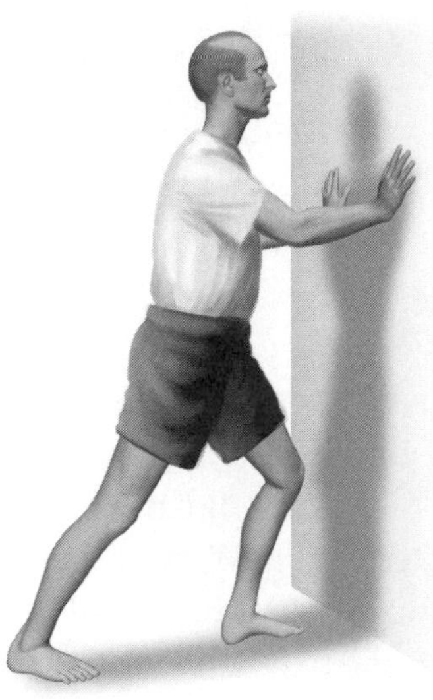

Calf stretch: Stand an arm's length from the wall. Lean into the wall. Place one leg forward with knee bent. Keep other leg back with knee straight and heel down. Keeping back straight, move hips toward the wall until you feel a stretch. Hold for 30 seconds. Relax. Repeat with the other leg.

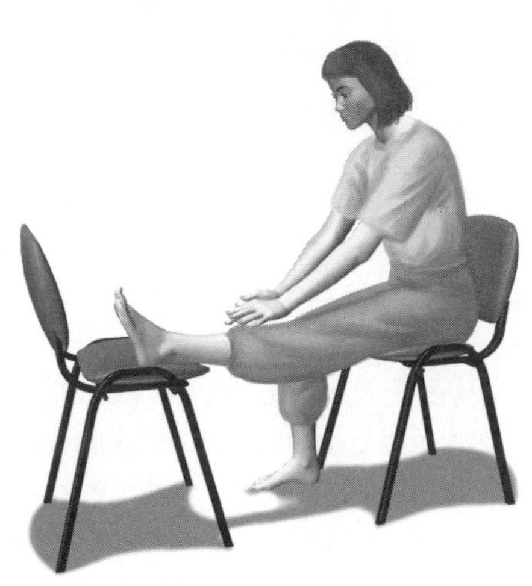

Hamstring stretch: Sit on a low table or a chair with one leg propped on another chair. Keep back straight. Without bending your knee, keep your back straight and lean forward until you feel a gentle pull in the back of your thigh. Hold the position for 30 seconds. Relax. Repeat with the other leg. (You can also do this exercise sitting on the floor with one leg out front and the other bent backward.)

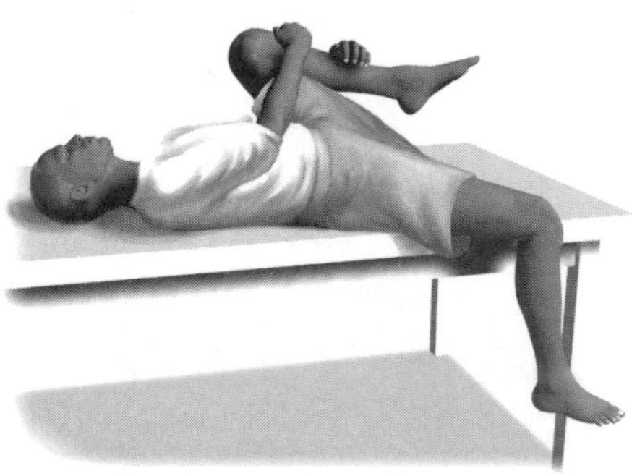

Upper-thigh stretch: Lie on a table or bed with one leg and hip as near the edge as possible and your lower leg hanging relaxed over the edge. Pull your other thigh and knee firmly toward your chest until your lower back flattens against the table. Hold for 30 seconds. Relax. Repeat with the other leg.

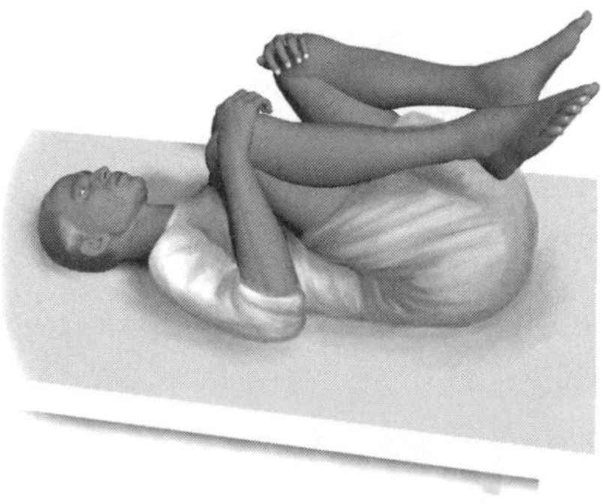

Lower-back stretch: Lie on a flat surface, such as the floor or a table, with your knees bent and feet flat on the surface. Grasp your knee and pull toward your shoulders. Stop when you feel a stretch in your lower back. Hold for 30 seconds. Relax. Repeat with the other leg.

Step 4: Emphasize aerobic fitness

Spend at least 30 minutes doing an aerobic activity you perceive as being fairly light to somewhat hard. If you've been inactive and are out of shape, begin with just 3 to 5 minutes at a very light pace. Then gradually increase your time by 1 to 3 minutes per session and your pace. Many people start with frenzied zeal and then quit when their muscles and joints become sore or injured.

After you've been active for a while and when you feel you're ready, gradually pick up the pace of your activity or increase the time you spend doing it by a few minutes each day. Instead of 30 minutes most days of the week, try aiming for 45 to 60 minutes.

When doing aerobic activities keep these suggestions in mind:

Mix your activities. Doing the same thing all of the time increases the chances that you'll become bored and quit being active. Think of activities beyond the common forms, such as canoeing, ballroom dancing or hiking. In addition, try to alternate among activities that emphasize lower- and upper-body fitness. Participating in a variety of activities also reduces your chance of injury to a specific muscle or overuse of a joint.

Be flexible. If you're overly tired or not feeling well, take a day or two off.

Listen to your body. A few minor aches and pains are bound to occur at times, but be aware of signs of overexertion or stress. (See "Avoiding injury" on page 117.)

Step 5: Build strength

At least twice a week, spend a few minutes doing exercises that help build strength. Greater muscle strength makes aerobic activity easier. A greater percentage of muscle than fat also increases the number of calories you use each day. In addition, stronger muscles, tendons and ligaments around your joints protect you against falls and fractures and reduce your risk of injury.

You build strength by working your muscles against your own body weight, large elastic bands or weighted objects (weights). The amount of weight or resistance you need to build muscle depends on your current strength. Choose a resistance that makes you feel as though you're working at a somewhat hard level on the

Perceived exertion scale (see page 107.)

At the start, light weights or low resistance and many repetitions help build muscle endurance. As you become stronger, gradually increase the weight or resistance or increase the number of repetitions.

Before lifting heavy weights, though, talk to your doctor. The strain of lifting heavy weights can cause a sharp increase in your blood pressure. This could possibly be dangerous if you have uncontrolled high blood pressure. Remember to breathe freely and to not hold your breath when you lift. Holding your breath during lifting can raise your blood pressure dramatically.

Simple strengthening exercises

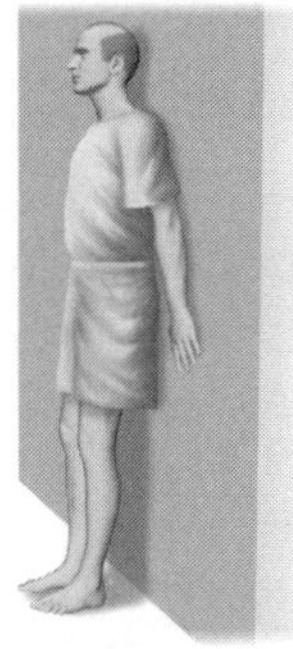

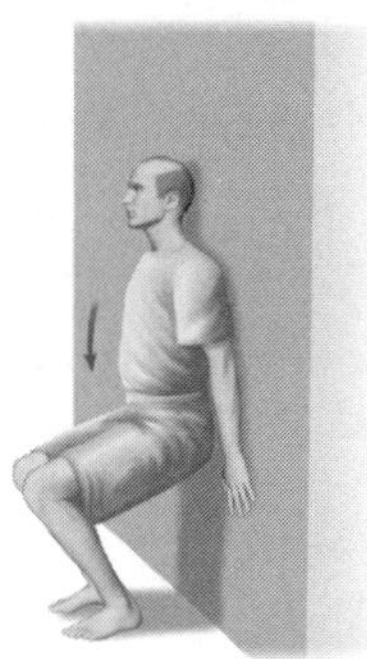

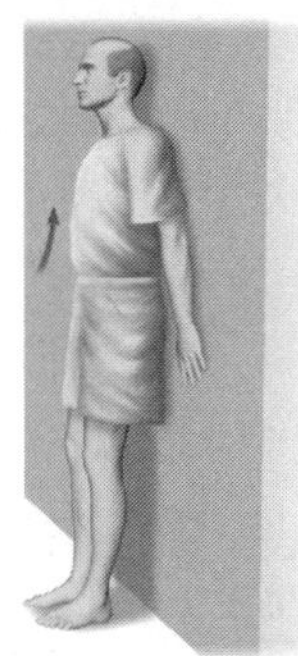

Wall slide: Stand with your heels about 12 inches (30.5 centimeters) from the wall. With your back against the wall, slowly slide down the surface until your knees are bent at a 45-degree angle. Slide back up to a standing position. This strengthens your quadriceps, improving walking and climbing strength.

Wall push-up: Face the wall and stand far enough away that you can place your palms on the wall with your elbows slightly bent. Slowly bend your elbows and lean toward the wall, supporting your weight with your arms. Straighten your arms and return to a standing position. This strengthens muscles in your arms and chest.

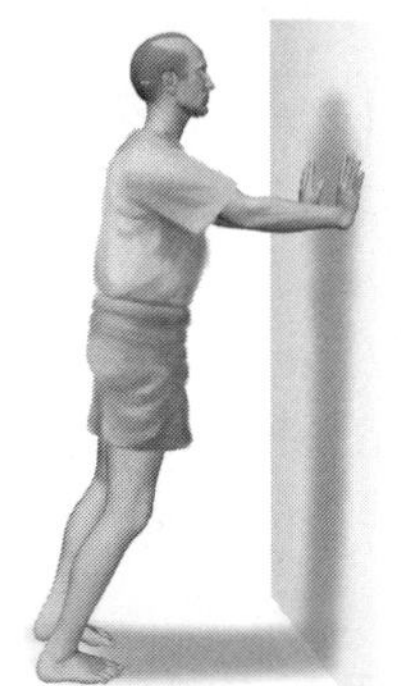

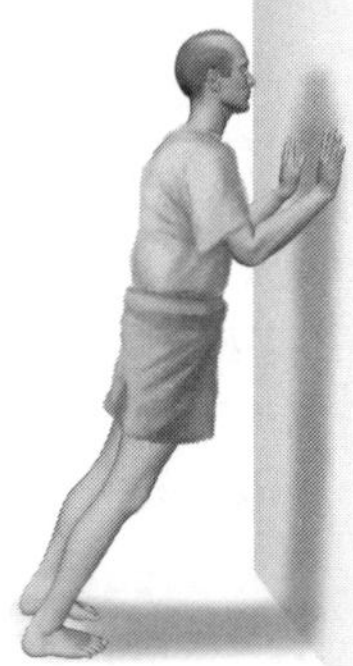

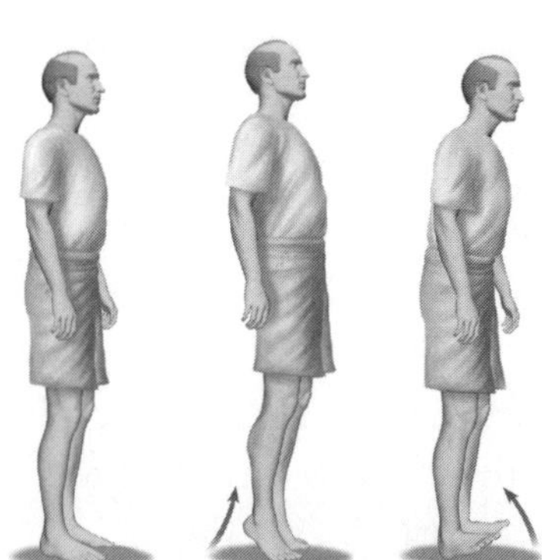

Toe and heel raise: Standing, rise up so that your weight is on your toes. Then rock back and shift your weight to your heels, lifting your toes off the ground. This strengthens your calf and lower leg muscles to improve your balance.

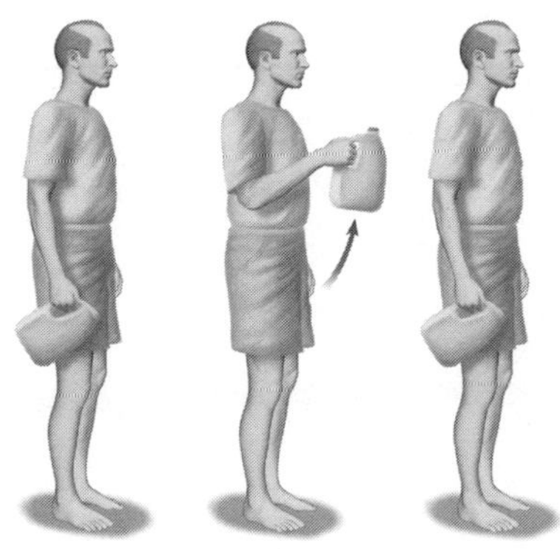

Arm curl: Stand with your feet shoulder-width apart. For resistance, hold a partially filled half-gallon milk jug. Flex your elbow until your hand reaches shoulder height. Hold, then lower your arm slowly. This tones your biceps and helps in carrying and lifting. Remember to keep your wrist rigid while lifting — don't bend or curl your wrist.

Step 6: Look for ways to stay motivated

Most people achieve a desirable level of fitness in 3 to 9 months. Your goal then is to maintain your fitness.

To keep up your motivation:

Track your progress. Measure your progress with a written log or diary. Seeing on paper how your fitness has improved can help keep you motivated to do more.

Adapt your activities. As you become more fit, fine-tune the intensity and duration of your activities.

Try new activities. Incorporating different and more challenging activities into your schedule will help keep it enjoyable. Also look for ways to include your family in your physical activities.

Avoiding injury

Injuries do occasionally happen during physical activity. However, you can reduce your risk of an injury by following these tips:

Drink plenty of water. Water helps maintain your normal body temperature and cools working muscles. To help replenish fluids that you lose, drink water before and after your activity.

Dress appropriately. Wear loosefitting, comfortable clothing that allows perspiration to escape from your body.

Warm up and cool down. Stretching before an aerobic activity prepares your body for the upcoming activity. Stretching afterward helps improve your flexibility. Warm up by walking before stretching. Avoid stretching cold muscles.

Be active regularly. Your risk of injury increases if you go back and forth between intense workouts and periods of inactivity.

Avoid start-and-stop activities. A controlled, continuous form of activity, such as walking or cycling, generally produces less risk of a muscle pull or other injury than do activities in which you start and stop frequently, such as basketball or tennis.

Don't compete. Avoid the physical and emotional intensity that often accompanies competitive sports.

Let food digest. Wait 2 to 3 hours after eating a large meal before being active. Digestion directs blood toward your digestive system and away from your heart.

Tailor your activity to the weather. When it's hot and humid, reduce your speed and distance. Or exercise early in the morning or later in the evening when it's cooler.

Avoid activity near heavy traffic. Breathing carbon monoxide given off by automobiles reduces the oxygen supply to your heart.

Know the warning signs. Seek immediate care if you experience any of these:

- Tightness in your chest
- Severe shortness of breath
- Chest pain or pain in your arms or jaw, often on the left side
- Fast, irregular heartbeats (palpitations)
- Dizziness, faintness or feeling sick to your stomach

Moderate activity shouldn't cause discomfort. Your breathing may be increased and you should feel like you're working. However, you shouldn't feel pain or experience exhaustion.

Wrap-up

Key points to remember:

- Regular physical activity can reduce your blood pressure by 5 to 10 mm Hg.
- Regular activity is more important than intensity.
- Get at least 30 minutes of moderately intense activity most, if not all, days of the week.
- Aerobic activity has the greatest effect on blood pressure.
- If time is a problem, look for ways to include more activity in your daily routine.

Chapter 8

Tobacco, alcohol and caffeine

Despite substantial progress in the effort to curtail the use of tobacco, millions of people continue to use it. And odds are that you're part of the great majority who at least occasionally has an alcoholic drink or regularly indulges in caffeinated coffee, tea or soft drinks.

Even if you're healthy, tobacco, alcohol and caffeine can raise your blood pressure to an unhealthy level. But if you have high blood pressure or you're at risk of it, you need to be especially alert to the effects that these substances can have on your blood pressure.

Tobacco and high blood pressure

Approximately one out of three people with high blood pressure smokes. Simply having high blood pressure puts you at increased risk of a heart attack or stroke. But if you have high blood pressure and you smoke, you're two to three times more likely to develop cardiovascular disease and three to five times more likely to die of a heart attack or heart failure than is someone who doesn't smoke. In addition, you're more than twice as likely to die of a stroke.

How smoking affects blood pressure

The nicotine in tobacco is what causes your blood pressure to increase shortly after you take that first puff. Nicotine, like many other chemicals in tobacco smoke, is picked up by tiny blood vessels in your lungs and distributed into your bloodstream. It takes only a few seconds for nicotine to reach your brain. Your brain reacts to nicotine by signaling your adrenal glands to release epinephrine (adrenaline). This powerful hormone narrows your blood vessels, forcing your heart to pump harder under higher pressure.

After smoking just two cigarettes, both systolic and diastolic pressures increase an average of about 10 millimeters of mercury (mm Hg). Your blood pressure remains at this increased level for about 30 minutes after you finish smoking. As the effects of the nicotine wear off, your blood pressure gradually decreases. However, if you smoke heavily, your blood pressure is at an increased level throughout most of the day. If you smoke, regularly measure your blood pressure at home. Let your doctor know if your home readings are higher than those during your checkups.

In addition to promoting the release of adrenaline, smoking has other damaging effects. The chemicals absorbed from tobacco smoke can affect the inner walls of your arteries, leaving them more susceptible to accumulation of cholesterol-containing fatty deposits (plaques) that narrow your arteries. Tobacco also triggers the release of hormones that cause your body to retain fluid. Both of these factors — narrowed arteries and increased fluid — can lead to high blood pressure.

Exposure to secondhand smoke also remains a serious health hazard. Each year in the United States, more than 50,000 nonsmokers die of heart disease caused by secondhand smoke. Exposure to secondhand smoke for as few as 5 minutes can cause changes in your arteries and heart. If you have other risk factors for heart disease, it's imperative that you avoid secondhand smoke. Even if you don't have other risk factors, exposure to secondhand smoke is hazardous to your health.

Why quitting is crucial

Stopping smoking may reduce your blood pressure by only a few points. But it's still important to stop. Here's why.

First, smoking interferes with some blood pressure medications, keeping them from working as well as they can, or sometimes from

Quitters do win

Many people continue to smoke because they figure they can't undo the damage already done to their bodies. Or they think that quitting is hopeless — they know too many smokers who tried to stop and failed. These assumptions are wrong.

Your body has an incredible ability to repair itself. By the end of your first nonsmoking year, your risk of heart attack is reduced by 50 percent, and after 5 years it's almost the same as that for people who have never smoked. In addition, after 10 to 15 years your risk of getting lung cancer and other cancers associated with tobacco use is about the same as that in people who never smoked.

It's true that most smokers aren't able to stop on their first attempt, particularly if they try to stop on their own. But stopping smoking is like learning anything else new. It often takes several attempts, and one bad experience shouldn't keep you from trying again. In fact, you can learn from previous attempts, increasing your chances for being successful in the future.

You can also enhance your chances for success by getting help from your doctor or by using a program that specializes in helping smokers stop.

It's true that many people gain weight after stopping smoking. But the negative consequences of the added weight are usually more than offset by the positive health benefits of stopping smoking.

working at all. Stopping smoking may increase the effectiveness of your medication.

Second, having high blood pressure puts you at increased risk of a heart attack, heart failure and stroke because of the damage it can cause to your heart, circulatory system and brain. Smoking also damages your arteries and produces the same cardiovascular risks as does high blood pressure. Therefore, when you combine high blood pressure with smoking, your odds for a heart attack, heart failure or stroke are much greater.

Research indicates that stopping smoking may raise blood pressure in some men. Why this occurs is unclear. However, stopping tobacco use yields enormous health benefits for most people.

You can work with your doctor to stay in control of your blood pressure as you stop smoking.

Breaking tobacco's grip

There's no one perfect plan for stopping smoking. Some people can simply stop and never smoke again. For others, quitting takes several tries and various approaches.

But you can stop — many people have. Following these steps can increase your chances for being successful.

Step 1: Do your homework. That way you'll know what to expect. You may experience physical withdrawal symptoms for at least 10 days. Common symptoms include irritability, anxiety and loss of concentration. Afterward, you may still have an urge to light up in familiar smoking situations, such as after a meal or while driving. These urges are generally very brief, but they can be very strong.

By knowing what to expect and having alternative activities planned, you'll be better prepared to handle the urges. These activities might include chewing gum after a meal or snacking on some carrot sticks or low-salt pretzels while driving to keep your hands busy.

Most relapses take place within 4 weeks after stopping smoking. Often, the relapse occurs both because of the power of nicotine addiction and because the smoker didn't have a well-conceived plan to avoid relapse situations.

Step 2: Set a stop date. Stopping cold turkey seems to work better than cutting down gradually. So carefully select a date to quit smoking. Don't try to stop when you know your stress level will be high.

Many smokers choose to stop during a relaxing vacation. One reason is that your routine changes on vacation, so it's easier to break free of smoking rituals than when you're at work or home.

Step 3: Talk with your doctor about medication and counseling. Nicotine is a highly addictive substance. Withdrawal from nicotine can produce irritability, anxiety and difficulty concentrating. Medications are available that can help lessen withdrawal symptoms and increase your chances of being successful (see "Medications to help you stop" on page 124).

Research indicates that medication can be effective for people who want to stop smoking — and that medication paired with counseling is even more effective. Ask your doctor about sources of counseling. In addition, many states and health organizations have telephone hot lines that provide advice and counseling.

Step 4: Tell others about your decision. Having the support of family, friends and co-workers can help you reach your goal more quickly. However, many smokers keep their plans to stop a secret. That's because they don't want to look like a failure if they go back to smoking.

Remember, it takes many people three or more tries before they're successful. So there's no reason to feel like a failure just because your effort may not work out this time. Enlisting the help of at least one person can enhance your chances of success.

Step 5: Start changing your routine. Before your stop date, cut down on the number of places you smoke. For instance, stop smoking in your car or in your home. This will help you become more comfortable in those places without smoking.

Step 6: Take one day at a time. On your stop day, quit completely. Each day, focus your attention on remaining tobacco-free.

Step 7: Avoid smoking situations. Change the situations in which you used to smoke. Leave the table immediately after meals if this is a time you used to light up. Take a walk instead. If you smoked while using the telephone, avoid long phone conversations or change the place where you talk. If you had a favorite smoking chair, avoid it.

To some degree, you'll become able to recognize when the urge to smoke is about to hit you. Before it hits, start doing something that makes smoking inconvenient, such as washing your car or mowing the lawn. Your smoking behavior is deeply ingrained and automatic. So you need to anticipate your reflex behavior and plan alternatives.

Step 8: Time each urge. Check your watch when a smoking urge hits. Most are short. Once you realize this, it's easier to resist. Remind yourself, "I can make it another few minutes, and then the urge will pass."

Use medications along with other strategies for quitting. Remember that medications are just one part of an overall plan to change your behavior.

Medications to help you stop

The medications listed below can reduce the difficult side effects of nicotine withdrawal and make stopping smoking easier. Use them according to your doctor's instructions or — in the case of over-the-counter (OTC) medications — according to the instructions on the label.

The nicotine medications listed below are used as temporary aids — usually for several weeks and almost always less than 6 months. The schedule for tapering off these medications will vary for each user. Ask your doctor for advice.

Nicotine patches. The Food and Drug Administration has approved four nicotine patches to help people stop smoking. Habitrol and ProStep are available with a physician's prescription. Nicoderm and Nicotrol are available without a prescription. The four patches deliver different amounts of nicotine.

A nicotine patch is placed on your skin. There it gradually releases nicotine into your body. This helps reduce nicotine cravings. Don't smoke while using a patch.

Patches may irritate your skin. To minimize the irritation, rotate the site of the patch and apply an OTC cortisone cream.

Nicotine gum. You can also purchase OTC nicotine gum. Two doses are available — 2 milligrams (mg) and 4 mg. The 4 mg product is recommended for heavier smokers.

Bite into the gum a few times, then "park" it between your cheek and gum. The lining of your mouth absorbs the nicotine that the gum releases. Nicotine gum can help to reduce the urge to smoke, much like the patch. Nicotine gum is also available by prescription. Again, don't smoke while using this medication.

Alcohol and high blood pressure

The best advice about alcohol is this — if you drink, do it in moderation.

Small amounts of alcohol don't seem to increase blood pressure. This is generally true even for people with high blood pressure. In fact, some evidence suggests that moderate drinking lowers the risk

Nicotine nasal spray. It helps you quit in the same way as the patch or gum, but instead you spray nicotine into your nose. There it's absorbed into your bloodstream through the lining of your nose, providing a quicker response to nicotine cravings than the other products provide. It's intended mainly for when you need a quick dose of nicotine and may be used with other nicotine replacement products or bupropion. The product is available only by prescription.

Nicotine inhaler. This medication is available only by prescription. The device looks like a plastic cigarette. You put the tip in your mouth and inhale. Puffing on the inhaler releases a nicotine vapor into your mouth, reducing your craving for nicotine. It also helps smokers who miss smoking's hand-to-mouth ritual.

Non-nicotine medications. Bupropion (Zyban) is a nonaddicting, non-nicotine medication approved by the FDA as a stop-smoking aid. It's not clear exactly how the drug works. One theory is that bupropion stimulates dopamine, a brain chemical that causes a feel-good response similar to that produced by nicotine and other drugs of addiction. Bupropion is available only by prescription.

Other non-nicotine medications may be used to treat tobacco dependence. According to guidelines issued in 2000 by the Department of Health and Human Services, these include clonidine and nortriptyline. However, the guidelines state that these drugs should be considered only if nicotine medications and bupropion are tried first and found to be ineffective. Clonidine and nortriptyline are also available by prescription only.

of heart attack by between 30 percent and 50 percent in middle-age people. It may also reduce the risk of developing blood clots that can lead to stroke. Moderate drinking can boost your production of high-density lipoprotein (HDL) cholesterol — the "good" form of cholesterol that helps protect your arteries from becoming narrowed or blocked by plaque.

Excessive alcohol is the problem. Drinking too much can increase your blood pressure and interfere with your medication. Heavy drinking is responsible for about 8 percent of all cases of high blood pressure in the United States.

Moderate drinking — less than you think?

Alcoholic drinks contain various amounts of ethanol — the more ethanol, the stronger the drink. For most men, moderate drinking is two drinks a day. Two drinks are equal to two 12-ounce (360-milliliter or mL) bottles of beer, two 5-ounce (150-mL) glasses of wine or two 1.5-ounce (45-mL) shot glasses of 80-proof liquor.

For women and small-framed men, moderate drinking is half that — one drink, or no more than half an ounce (15 mL) of ethanol daily. The amount is less because women metabolize alcohol differently than men do, and people with smaller builds have smaller volumes of blood, which results in higher concentrations of ethanol. For men and women age 65 and older, moderate drinking is one drink a day.

Remember that the effects of drinking on health are still being studied. Even moderate drinking may not be good for some people. Be sure to consult with your doctor about how drinking affects your overall health and blood pressure.

Too much + too soon = too high

If you drink too much alcohol and you want to cut back, it's best to gradually reduce how much you drink over a period of 1 to 2 weeks.

People who drink heavily and suddenly stop consuming alcohol can develop severe high blood pressure that lasts for several days. That's because when you suddenly remove alcohol from your blood, your body releases large amounts of epinephrine (adrenaline), which causes your blood pressure to rise sharply.

If you have high blood pressure and you drink more than a moderate amount of alcohol, talk with your doctor about the safest and most successful way to limit or avoid alcohol.

How alcohol affects blood pressure

Exactly how excessive alcohol — more than a moderate amount — increases blood pressure is unknown. One theory is that it triggers the release of epinephrine (adrenaline) and other hormones that narrow your blood vessels or cause you to retain more sodium and water. Excessive drinking is also associated with poor nutrition, which could deplete your levels of calcium and magnesium. Low levels of these minerals are associated with higher blood pressure.

However, it's clear that reducing your consumption of alcohol can reduce your blood pressure. Excessive drinkers who cut back to moderate levels of alcohol consumption can lower their systolic blood pressure by about 5 mm Hg and their diastolic pressure about 3 mm Hg.

Combining a nutritious diet with reduced alcohol use can produce an even larger reduction — a drop of about 10 mm Hg in systolic pressure and 7 mm Hg in diastolic pressure. One reason for this effect is that people who consume too much alcohol generally don't get adequate amounts of nutrients that help control blood pressure, such as potassium, calcium and magnesium.

People on blood pressure medication who limit alcohol also tend to be more diligent about taking their medication. When influenced by alcohol, you may forget to take your pills or take them improperly.

Alcohol and blood pressure medications

If you take medication, you may need to pay careful attention to when or how you consume alcohol. Alcohol can interfere with the effectiveness of some blood pressure medications and increase their side effects.

If you mix alcohol with a beta blocker, which relaxes your blood vessels and slows your heart rate, you may feel lightheaded or faint — especially if you're overheated or if you stand suddenly. You can experience the same symptoms if you drink alcohol near the time you take an angiotensin-converting enzyme (ACE) inhibitor, which widens your blood vessels, or certain calcium antagonists, which can slow your heart rate. If you do feel dizzy or faint, sit until the feeling passes. Drinking water also may help.

In general, any medication that causes drowsiness shouldn't be taken with alcohol. Read the label before you decide to consume alcohol and listen to your body. If you feel lightheaded or depressed after a drink or two, talk with your doctor about how much alcohol you can safely drink and when.

Caffeine and high blood pressure

Found in coffee, tea, soft drinks and chocolate, caffeine is a mild stimulant. Caffeine can fight fatigue, boost your concentration and lighten your mood. Tea also contains flavonoids and other antioxidants that may contribute to the reduced cardiovascular disease reported in some tea drinkers.

But if you use too much — something that's easy to do — caffeine can leave you jittery, cause your hands to tremble and possibly increase your blood pressure. The amount of caffeine in two to three cups of coffee — 200 to 250 mg — has been shown to raise systolic pressure 3 to 14 mm Hg and diastolic pressure 4 to 13 mm Hg in people without high blood pressure.

How caffeine affects blood pressure

Caffeine's influence on blood pressure is a topic of debate. Some studies have found that people who consume caffeine regularly throughout the day have a higher average blood pressure than if they didn't consume any. However, many studies report that regular consumers of caffeine develop a tolerance to the stimulant. And after awhile, it doesn't have any effect on their blood pressure.

Among people who don't consume caffeine regularly or who consume more than they're used to, caffeine can cause a temporary but sharp rise in blood pressure.

Cut back slowly

If you plan to reduce caffeine, the best way is to taper the amount you drink over several weeks. This will help you avoid headaches and other side effects that can result when you drastically reduce your use of caffeine.

Calculating your caffeine intake

If you have high blood pressure, limit caffeine to about 200 milligrams (mg) daily. Here are some common sources of caffeine and the amount of caffeine they contain:

Source	Caffeine (mg)
Coffee, ¾ cup (6 fl oz/180 mL)	
Brewed, drip	103
Instant	57
Decaffeinated, brewed and instant	2
Espresso (single)	
Regular	100
Decaffeinated	5
Tea, ¾ cup (6 fl oz/180 mL)	
Black, brewed 3 minutes	40
Instant	30
Decaffeinated	1
Soft drinks, 1½ cups (12 fl oz/360 mL)	
Cola type, regular and diet	31 to 70
Noncola type	0 to 55
Chocolate	
Cocoa, dry powder, 1 tbsp.	10
Baking chocolate, 1 oz (30 g)	25
Chocolate milk, 1 cup (8 fl oz/250 mL)	10
Milk chocolate bar, 1½ oz (45 g)	10

Source: *Bowes and Church's Food Values of Portions Commonly Used*, 1998.

Exactly what causes this spike in blood pressure is uncertain. Some researchers suggest that caffeine narrows your blood vessels by blocking the effects of adenosine (uh-DEN-uh-seen), a hormone that helps keep them widened. Caffeine may also stimulate the adrenal gland to release more cortisol and adrenaline.

As a precaution, many doctors advise people with high blood pressure to limit daily caffeine intake to no more than two cups of coffee, three or four cups of tea or two to four cans of caffeinated soda.

In addition, avoid caffeine right before activities that naturally increase your blood pressure, such as exercise or hard physical labor.

Limiting caffeine is also good for your general health. Depending on your sensitivity to caffeine, even a couple of cups of coffee can affect your:

Nervous system. Too much caffeine can make you nervous, anxious or irritable. It also can worsen panic attacks and cause insomnia.

Digestive system. Caffeine can produce heartburn, constipation, diarrhea and gastrointestinal upset or can irritate existing stomach ulcers.

Bladder. Caffeine can cause bladder irritation in some people. It's also a mild diuretic, causing you to urinate more.

Wrap-up

Key points to remember:

- If you have high blood pressure and you smoke, your risk of death from a heart attack or heart failure is at least three times higher, and your risk of death from stroke is at least two times higher than if you didn't smoke.
- Medications designed to reduce nicotine withdrawal can help you stop smoking. Specialized treatment programs, telephone hot lines and your doctor can provide advice and support.
- Eight percent of all cases of high blood pressure are due to excessive use of alcohol.
- For many people, moderate alcohol use doesn't appear to affect blood pressure.
- Alcohol may increase the side effects of some high blood pressure medications.
- Caffeine can cause a temporary but sharp rise in blood pressure in some people.
- If you have high blood pressure, limit caffeine to two cups of coffee, three or four cups of tea or two to four cans of caffeinated soda daily.

Chapter 9

Managing stress

Consider a common belief: If you lead a stressful life or you're a Type A personality — competitive, intense, impatient — you're destined to have high blood pressure. This is not entirely true. There are many Type A individuals with normal blood pressure, just as there are relaxed people with high blood pressure.

Stress can increase your blood pressure temporarily. When you're scared, nervous or under a tight deadline, your blood pressure may increase. But in most cases, once you begin to relax, your blood pressure goes back down again.

If you have high blood pressure, simply reducing your stress level may not completely lower your blood pressure. But managing stress is important for other reasons. Less stress often results in the following:

Better control of blood pressure. The temporary increases in blood pressure caused by stress can make your high blood pressure more difficult to manage. When you're under less stress, lifestyle changes and medications may work more effectively.

A more positive attitude. Stress can interfere with and dampen your enthusiasm to take control of your blood pressure. It's easier to be physically active, eat a healthy diet, lose weight and limit alcohol when you're relaxed and happy.

There are many ways to manage stress. You may want to experiment with some different techniques until you find those stress relievers that fit your lifestyle and daily routine.

What is stress?

Think of stress as a spice. Too little spice results in a bland-tasting meal. Too much spice can make you sick. But when you use the correct amount, spice enhances flavor. Stress works in much the same way.

Stress can be positive or negative

Stress is what you experience when emotional, physical or environmental demands challenge or exceed your personal resources and ability to cope effectively. But it's important to remember that stress isn't these various outside influences. Rather, it's how you respond to these influences.

Positive stress. This form of stress provides a feeling of excitement and opportunity. You feel confident when approaching a situation. Among athletes, positive stress often helps them perform better in competition than in practice. Other examples of positive stressors may include a new job or the birth of a child.

Negative stress. This stress occurs when you feel out of control or under constant pressure. You may have trouble concentrating on a project. You may feel isolated from others. Family, finances, work and isolation are common causes of negative stress.

Despite this positive-negative distinction, physiologically your body tends to respond the same way to either kind of stress. It's how you perceive the stress that makes it positive or negative for you. Stress is therefore highly individualized. Some people cope well with difficult or tense situations. Others melt under pressure. In addition, what's a stressor for one person may not cause stress for another.

Major stress can result from minor aggravations that accumulate over time. You can benefit from responding to those aggravations right away and learning to manage stress on a daily basis.

The stress response

When dealing with a frightful event or an ongoing tension in your life, your body's physical response to any stressor is similar to a physical threat. Your body gears up to face the challenge (fight) or gathers enough strength to move out of trouble's way (flight).

This fight-or-flight response results from the release of an assortment of hormones that cause your body to shift into overdrive. Among them are the hormones epinephrine (adrenaline) and cortisol, which cause your heart to beat faster and your blood pressure to increase.

Other physical changes also occur. More blood and nutrients are sent to your brain and muscles, and less to your skin. That's why you may look pale during moments of fright or high stress. Your body also releases fibrin, a protein that makes your blood clot more easily. In a physical attack, this would help slow or stop bleeding from a wound.

Your nervous system also springs into action. Your pupils dilate to enhance your vision. Your facial muscles tense up to make you look more intimidating. And you perspire more to cool your body.

Your body has many ways of letting you know when it's under too much stress. You may become discouraged, irritable, cynical, emotional or even reclusive. All of these emotions affect how you think, feel and act. However, these changes can sometimes be easy to miss because they may sneak up gradually, over a long time.

The physical signs and symptoms aren't as easy to ignore. They may include a headache, stomach upset, insomnia, fatigue and frequent illness. You may find yourself reverting to nervous habits, such as biting your nails or smoking. You might even turn to alcohol or drugs.

Stress and blood pressure

The hormones epinephrine (adrenaline) and cortisol released during periods of stress increase blood pressure by narrowing your blood vessels and increasing your heart rate. The increase in blood pressure caused by stress varies, depending on your level of stress and how your body copes with stress. In some people, stress causes only a slight increase in blood pressure. In others, stress can produce extreme jumps in blood pressure.

The effects of acute stress are usually only temporary. However, if you experience stress regularly, the increases in blood pressure that it produces can over time damage your arteries, heart, brain, kidneys and eyes — just as with persistent high blood pressure. This cumulative effect of stress often goes unrecognized until it manifests itself as a serious health problem.

Strategies for relieving stress

It's one thing to be aware of stress in your daily life. And it's another thing to know what to do about it.

Stress becomes a problem whenever the demands of your environment threaten to overcome or actually exceed your ability to cope. There are three basic ways that you can respond — change your environment, change how you cope, or change both. Following are ways to accomplish these three goals.

Lifestyle changes

Making some changes in your normal routine can lessen your stress load. They include:

Get organized. Keep a written schedule of your daily activities so that you're not faced with conflicts or last-minute rushes to get to an appointment or activity on time. Take on tasks — especially those that seem most stressful — at the time of day when you feel your best. For some people, that time is morning. For others, it's afternoon or evening.

Simplify your schedule. Try to adopt a more relaxed pace. Set aside your can-do mentality and learn how to say no to added responsibilities that you don't feel up to tackling. Ask others to lend a hand.

Relieve work-related stress. Frustration with your job can be a major source of stress. To relieve this source of stress, look for ways to upgrade your job performance and satisfaction. Learn ways to resolve conflict with co-workers. Also create a career plan with short-term and long-term goals. Figure out what skills you'll need to meet your goals and create a plan to develop those skills.

Build a financial cushion. If you become unemployed, take a cut in pay or face an unexpected large expense, your stress levels could rise overnight. Having some extra cash in the bank is one way to cope. Begin to create a financial cushion now. See if you can take at least 10 percent of every paycheck and deposit that money in a savings account or low-risk investment. Knowing that you have a financial cushion can soften the blow of money-related stress.

Exercise. In addition to helping control your blood pressure, exercise tends to counter the adverse effects of stress. Exercise 30 to 60 minutes most days of the week.

Eat well. A varied diet provides the right mix of nutrients that can help keep your immune system and other body systems working well. A healthy diet emphasizes grains, fruits, vegetables and low-fat dairy products.

Get plenty of sleep. When you're refreshed, you're better able to tackle the next day's problems. Going to sleep and awakening at a consistent time each day can help you sleep well. A bedtime ritual, such as taking a warm bath, reading or listening to music can aid in falling asleep.

Stress and your overall health

Stress is thought to play a role in several illnesses. When your heart rate increases, you become at greater risk of chest pain (angina) and irregularities in your heart rhythm (arrhythmia). Surges in your heart rate and blood pressure can also trigger a heart attack or damage your heart muscle or coronary arteries. The blood-clotting protein fibrin released when you're under stress also puts you at increased risk of blood clots.

The hormone cortisol is released during stress and it may suppress your immune system. There is evidence this suppression may make you more susceptible to infectious diseases, including upper respiratory viral infections such as cold or flu.

Stress can also trigger headaches and may worsen asthma and intestinal problems. It may also lengthen the time needed for wound healing.

Change your act. Observe your posture and behavior when you feel overly stressed. You might find that you slump your shoulders, breathe in a more shallow way or reduce your activity level. Times of high stress may even lead you to neglect your appearance or avoid people.

One stress management technique is to act the part of a confident, relaxed person. You can do this even when you don't feel particularly relaxed or confident. Pay attention to your posture, breathe deeply, keep exercising and stay in contact with people. Even getting a haircut, manicure or new outfit might help. Over time, changing your physical presence could change your emotional state and promote your confidence.

Give yourself an occasional break. Get away from your regular routine and the stresses in your life. Take a vacation, even if it's just for a weekend — and plan it so that you leave your stressful problems behind. Take time to see a movie or enjoy a relaxing meal out. During the workday, take short breaks to stretch, walk, breathe deeply and relax.

Maintain good social relationships. Friends and family provide a release valve that lets you vent your frustrations, but also can give you helpful advice that points you toward solutions. However, avoid talking with friends and family members who tend to be negative about everything and who foster bad feelings. Try to surround yourself with positive, supportive people.

Change your thinking. Monitor your self-talk to tone down your critical or negative feelings. Self-talk refers to all of the things that you say to yourself — all of the thoughts that run through your head. For example, instead of "I should never make a mistake," tell yourself "Everyone makes mistakes, and I will be more careful next time." This approach can reduce negative feelings.

Schedule worry time. Setting aside time for problem solving can keep your worries from adding up. Devote a half-hour each day to work on solutions to problems. If a worry crops up outside of worry time, write it down and worry about it later.

Look for humor. Laughter is an upper. It releases chemicals in your brain that ease pain and enhance a feeling of well-being.

Laughter stimulates your heart, lungs and muscles. Just 20 seconds of laughter produces an oxygen exchange that equals about 3 minutes of aerobic exercise. Find a movie that makes you laugh out loud or books by authors you enjoy.

Relaxation techniques

Not all stress is avoidable. There are certain events in life that you can't prevent, such as getting stuck in an unexpected traffic jam. But you can reduce the emotional and physical toll these events can take.

When you're feeling stressed, take a few minutes to relax your body and clear your head. The following exercises are designed to help you do this. However, keep in mind that relaxation doesn't happen automatically. To develop this skill, you need to practice it daily. If you're not successful, see a qualified behavioral health care professional.

Deep breathing. Unlike children, most adults breathe from their chest. Each time you breathe in, your chest expands, and each time you breathe out, it contracts. Children, however, generally breathe from their diaphragm, the muscle that separates the chest from the abdomen.

Deep breathing from your diaphragm — which adults can relearn — is relaxing. It also exchanges more carbon dioxide for oxygen to give you more energy. This kind of breathing can act on centers in your brain that lower blood pressure. (See "Taking a breather" on page 138.)

A medical device called Resperate is designed to help lower blood pressure with deep breathing. The device includes an elastic belt with a respiration sensor, headphones and a small unit that looks like a portable CD player. The device analyzes your breathing pattern and then creates two distinct tones to guide your inhalation and exhalation. The goal is to lengthen your exhalation and to slow your breathing to fewer than 10 breaths per minute. The device is available over-the-counter.

Muscle tension exercises. When tension mounts, it can tighten your muscles, especially in your shoulders. To relieve the tightness, roll your shoulders, raising them toward your ears. Then relax your shoulders.

To reduce neck tension, move your head gently in a circle going clockwise, then counterclockwise. To relieve tension in your back and torso, reach toward the ceiling and do side bends. For foot and leg tension, draw circles in the air with your feet while flexing your toes.

Daily stretching exercises also help reduce muscle tension.

Guided imagery. Also known as visualization, this method of relaxation involves lying quietly and picturing yourself in a pleasant and peaceful setting. You experience the setting with all of your senses,

Taking a breather

Here's an exercise to help you practice deep, relaxed breathing.

1. Wear comfortable clothes that are loose around your waist. Lie on your back on a bed, a recliner or a padded floor. You can also sit in a chair if you prefer.
2. Place your feet slightly apart. Rest one hand on your abdomen near your navel. Put your other hand on your chest. If you're sitting, place your feet flat on the floor, relax your shoulders and place your hands in your lap or at your side.
3. Inhale through your nose, if you can, because this filters and warms the air. Exhale through your mouth.
4. Concentrate on your breathing for a few minutes and notice which hand is rising with each breath.
5. Gently exhale most of the air in your lungs.
6. Inhale while slowly counting to four, about 1 second per count. As you inhale, slightly raise your abdomen about an inch (2.5 centimeters). You should be able to feel the movement with your hand. Don't move your chest or pull your shoulders up.
7. As you breathe in, imagine the air flowing to all parts of your body, supplying you with cleansing and energizing oxygen.
8. Pause for a second with the air in your lungs. Then slowly exhale, again counting to four. You'll feel your abdomen slowly fall as your diaphragm relaxes. Imagine the tension flowing out of you.
9. Pause for a moment. Then begin again and repeat this exercise for 1 to 2 minutes, until you feel better. If you experience lightheadedness, shorten the length or depth of your breathing.

A sample lesson in relaxation

This stress reliever involves blocking out the world and concentrating specifically on relaxing your body.

1. Sit or lie in a comfortable position and close your eyes. To allow for natural circulation, uncross your arms and legs. Allow your jaw to drop and your eyelids to become relaxed and heavy but not tightly closed.

2. Mentally scan your body. Start with your toes and work slowly up to your legs, buttocks, torso, arms, hands, fingers, neck, head and face. As you do this, tighten each set of muscles and hold them for a count of five before relaxing. As the muscles relax, imagine the tension melting away.

3. During this exercise, allow your mind to become peaceful and calm. Thoughts will flow through your mind. Let them come and go without dwelling on any of them.

4. Suggest to yourself that you're relaxed and calm, that your hands are heavy and warm — or cool if you're hot — that your heart is beating calmly and that you're at perfect peace. Allow a sense of relaxation to flow through your body.

5. Breathe slowly, regularly and deeply during the exercise.

6. Once you're relaxed, imagine you're in a favorite place or in a spot of great beauty and stillness.

7. After 5 to 10 minutes, gradually rouse yourself.

as if you were actually there. Imagine the sounds, scents, warmth, breezes and colors of this comforting place. The messages your brain receives as you experience these senses help your body to relax.

Meditation. It involves sitting in a comfortable position and repeating a sound or word for 20 minutes, usually twice a day. Your goal is to clear your mind of all distracting thoughts and reach a restful state. One study found that people with high blood pressure who practiced meditation not only reduced their blood pressure, but also lowered their heart rate and widened their arteries.

Professional help

Sometimes, life's stresses can pile up and become more than you can deal with on your own. When they do, consider getting help from your doctor or a qualified behavioral counselor. Some people believe that seeking outside help is a sign of weakness. Nothing could be further from the truth. It takes strength of character to admit you need help.

Learning how to control your stress won't guarantee you a relaxed life, good health and normal blood pressure. Unexpected problems will still occur. But having the tools to deal with stress can make those problems easier to overcome — and your blood pressure easier to control.

Wrap-up

Key points to remember:

- Stress can increase your blood pressure temporarily and aggravate existing high blood pressure.
- Over time, the physical effects of stress can be damaging to your health.
- Although reducing stress may not completely lower your blood pressure, it can make your blood pressure easier to control.
- Lifestyle changes, relaxation techniques and professional help can help you avoid or better manage stress and reduce health risks.

Chapter 10

Staying in control

High blood pressure isn't an illness you can treat and then ignore. It's a condition that you need to manage for the rest of your life. This can sometimes be difficult because you can't feel or see anything wrong. With many diseases, such as arthritis or allergies, symptoms motivate you to seek treatment. You feel the flaring pain of arthritic joints or you experience the sneezing, itchy eyes and cough of an allergy. You want to control your disease or condition because you want symptoms to go away.

Lack of symptoms is why people with high blood pressure often don't take steps to treat their disease. It's also why only about 25 percent of Americans with high blood pressure have it under control.

Managing high blood pressure — measuring your blood pressure at home, taking your medications properly, maintaining a proper diet and exercise program, making regular visits to your doctor — is essential. It can significantly increase your chances for living a longer, healthier life, despite high blood pressure.

Home monitoring

Your doctor's office isn't the only place to measure your blood pressure. You can do it yourself at home. Blood pressure monitors are available at medical supply stores and many pharmacies. They're not difficult to use — especially once you've had a little practice.

If your blood pressure is well controlled, checking it two or three days a month is often adequate. Take and record two readings in the morning and two in the evening on a day that you're working, and two pairs of readings on a day that you're relaxing. If your blood pressure isn't well controlled, ask your doctor how often you should measure it.

For purposes of home monitoring, staying in control means an average systolic pressure of 134 millimeters of mercury (mm Hg) or less and an average diastolic pressure of 84 mm Hg or less. This is equivalent to a systolic pressure of 139 mm Hg or less and a diastolic pressure of 89 mm Hg or less in the doctor's office.

Benefits of home monitoring

Measuring your blood pressure at home can help:

Track your treatment. Because high blood pressure has no symptoms, the only way to make sure lifestyle changes or your medications are working is to check your blood pressure regularly. Monitoring your blood pressure at home gives you essential information to share with the people who provide your health care.

Promote better control. When you take the initiative to measure your own blood pressure, this responsible act tends to rub off on other areas. It can give you added incentive to eat a better diet, increase your activity level and take your medication properly.

Identify white-coat hypertension. For some people, simply going to a doctor's office increases their blood pressure. Home monitoring can help determine whether you have true high blood pressure or white-coat hypertension.

Save money. Home monitoring saves you the cost of going to your doctor's office to have your blood pressure taken. This is especially true when you first start to take medication or your doctor adjusts your medication. In these cases, frequent measurements help to ensure better control.

Types of blood pressure monitors

Not all blood pressure monitors are the same. Some are easier to use, others are more reliable, and some are inaccurate and a waste of money. To get an accurate reading, place an appropriately sized cuff around your upper arm. It's important that the cuff fits you properly. The inflatable bladder in the cuff should encircle 80 percent to 100 percent of your upper arm and reach three-fourths of the way from your elbow to your shoulder. Ideally, the cuff will have a D-ring to help with closure. Have your doctor or other health care professional measure your arm to determine the appropriate size cuff for you. This is particularly important if you have a large upper arm.

Blood pressure monitors are available in these forms:

Mercury-column models. These monitors, which look like oversized thermometers, once were the standard. Due to safety concerns about mercury poisoning and environmental concerns over disposal of mercury, they're being phased out.

Aneroid models. These monitors feature a round dial. Each increment on the dial corresponds to 2 millimeters of mercury. Blood pressure is indicated by a needle on the face of the dial.

Health care professionals often recommend aneroid models because they're inexpensive and easy to transport. In addition, some dials are extra-large for easier reading and some models have a built-in stethoscope for easier use.

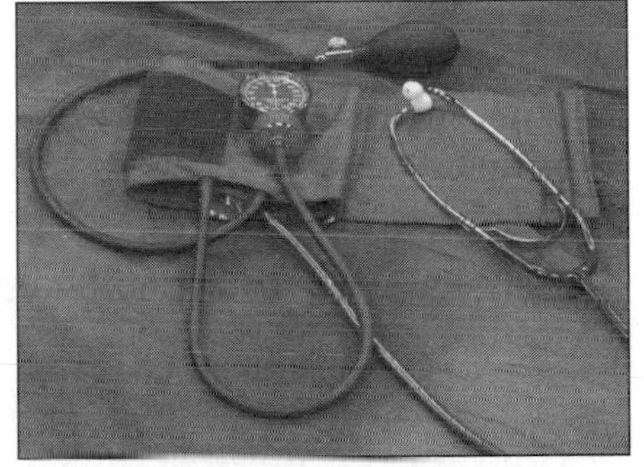

An aneroid blood pressure monitor includes a cuff, a rubber bulb to inflate the cuff, a stethoscope to listen for your pulse and a gauge on which to read your pressure.

A disadvantage is that once a year you need to verify the monitor's accuracy by comparing it to a standard. You can do this by taking your monitor with you to your doctor's office. If the reading is more than 3 millimeters off, you should replace the unit.

Standard aneroid monitors aren't recommended if you have trouble hearing or if you have poor dexterity in your hands. These monitors require that you to listen for your heartbeat and the sounds of blood passing through the artery — called auscultation. They also require use of a stethoscope and bulb pump.

Electronic models. Also referred to as digital monitors, these models are the most popular and the easiest to use. Electronic models are also the most expensive device for home monitoring, though they continue to decline in price.

Electronic blood pressure monitors generally require that you do just two things — put the cuff on your arm and push a button. The cuff automatically inflates with air and then slowly deflates. Your blood pressure measurement is displayed on a screen.

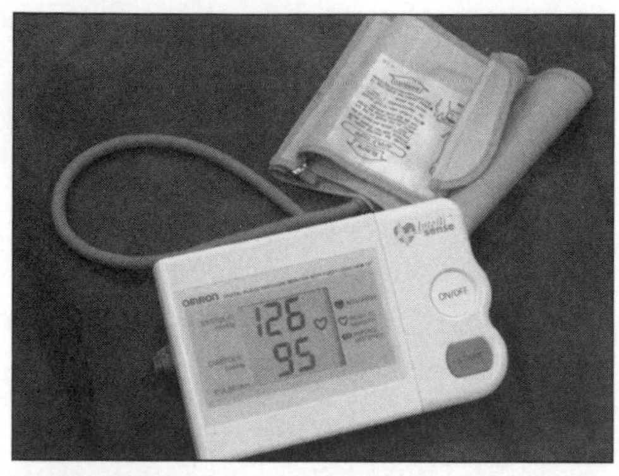

Electronic blood pressure monitors are the most popular and the easiest to use.

As with aneroid models, you need to check the electronic monitor's accuracy at least once a year. Electronic monitors are also easier to damage.

If you have an irregular heart rhythm, check with your doctor before buying an electronic monitor. It may give you an inaccurate reading.

Contrary to mercury-column and aneroid models, electronic monitors detect motion in the artery wall — called oscillometry — rather than sound. For a small number of people, aneroid and electronic monitors may not give exactly the same measurements.

Finger or wrist models. To make blood pressure monitors more compact and easier to use, some manufacturers have produced models that measure blood pressure in your wrist or finger, instead of your upper arm. To get an accurate reading with either of these models, it's very important that your hand and wrist be at heart level. Unfortunately, the technology of finger monitors hasn't caught up with their simplicity of use. Avoid them because they're inaccurate. And the wrist monitors are difficult to calibrate.

Home monitoring tips

Learning to take your blood pressure correctly takes practice and a little training. After you purchase a blood pressure monitor, take it with you to your doctor's office.

In addition to making sure the device works properly, your doctor or nurse can help you learn how to use it. Some medical facilities also offer classes in taking blood pressure. Keep in mind that if you have an irregular heart rhythm, getting an accurate reading will be more difficult.

To accurately measure your blood pressure:

- Don't measure your blood pressure right after you get up in the morning. Wait until after you've been active for an hour or more. If you exercise after you awaken, check your blood pressure before you exercise.
- Take it before you eat or wait at least a half-hour after you've eaten, smoked or used caffeine or alcohol. Food, tobacco, caffeine and alcohol can increase your pressure.
- Go to the bathroom first. A full bladder increases your blood pressure slightly.
- Sit quietly for about 5 minutes before taking a reading.
- Remember that your blood pressure varies throughout the day. Readings are often a little higher in the morning. Your mood also can affect your blood pressure. If you've had a difficult day, don't be alarmed if your blood pressure reflects it.
- Use proper technique. Follow these 10 steps listed below. If you have an electronic device, some steps won't apply, so ask your doctor for additional instructions.

Step 1: Sit comfortably. Keep your legs and ankles uncrossed and your back supported against the back of a chair. Rest your arm at heart level on a table or the arm of a chair. If you're right-handed, you may find it easier to measure pressure in your left arm and vice versa. Be consistent with which arm you use.

Step 2: If you use an aneroid model, find your pulse in the arm on which you'll place the cuff so you'll know where to place the stethoscope. Do this by pressing firmly on the inside of your elbow, above the bend. If you can't find it, you may be pressing either too hard or too soft.

Step 3: Wrap the cuff around your bare arm. Place the cuff about 2 inches (5 centimeters) above your elbow bend. The inflatable portion of the cuff should wrap all the way around your arm and fit snugly. Different sized cuffs are available. Make sure yours fits properly. A cuff with a D-ring is easier to use.

Step 4: If you're using an aneroid model, place the earpieces of the stethoscope into your ears, with the earpieces facing forward.

Place the diaphragm or flat side of the stethoscope where you located your pulse, putting the diapragm firmly and directly over your main artery, just under the lower 1 to 2 inches of the cuff. If your monitor has a built-in stethoscope (sometimes marked with an arrow), place the diaphragm over the area where you located your pulse. If the arterial sounds aren't clearly heard, place the bell side of the stethoscope below the lower edge of the cuff.

Step 5: Put the gauge or electronic screen where you can easily read it. Make sure it registers at zero before you inflate the cuff.

Step 6: Using the hand of your uncuffed arm, squeeze the hand bulb repeatedly to pump air into the cuff. Inflate the cuff about 30 millimeters (mm) above your usual systolic pressure (upper number), then stop. You shouldn't hear your pulse when listening through the stethoscope.

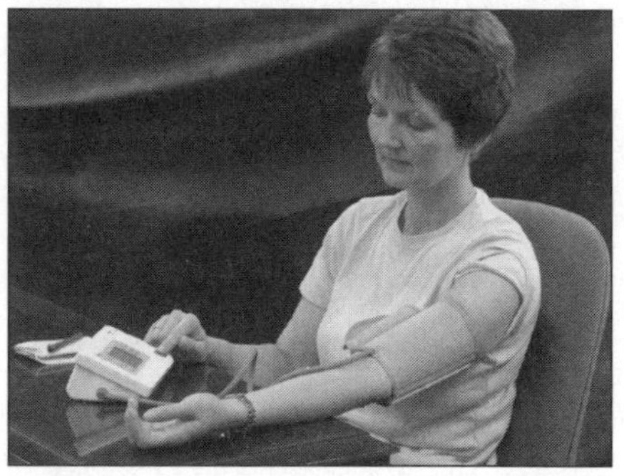

Using an electronic model involves sitting with your arm at heart level, placing the cuff around your upper arm, relaxing and pressing a button to inflate the cuff and get a reading.

Step 7: Turn the release valve and slowly deflate the cuff at 2 to 3 mm per second. Watch the gauge and if you have an aneroid model, listen carefully. When you hear the first tapping sound of your pulse, note the reading on the gauge. If the gauge's needle jerks slightly, use the lowest reading. This is your systolic pressure.

Step 8: Continue deflating the cuff. When the pulse sounds stop, note the gauge's reading. This is your diastolic pressure. For some people, the pulse doesn't disappear, but it will fade noticeably.

Video demonstration of home monitoring

Visit the High Blood Pressure Center on MayoClinic.com to see a video on how to use home blood pressure monitors. The video shows the proper technique for both aneroid and automatic (digital) monitors. To view the video, go to *www.MayoClinic.com,* click High Blood Pressure Center and look for the link "How to monitor your own blood pressure" in the "Take Control" section.

That sudden drop in sound marks the diastolic pressure. Then release the valve completely.

Step 9: Wait 2 minutes after the first reading and repeat the procedure to check for accuracy. If you have trouble getting consistent readings, check with your doctor. The problem may be your technique or equipment. Also contact your doctor if you notice an unusual or persistent increase in your blood pressure.

Step 10: Keep a log of your blood pressure readings. Along with each reading, include date and time. Show your log to your doctor during your next appointment. Below is a sample log.

Date	Time	Systolic pressure	Diastolic pressure	Pulse	Medication changes/comments

Using your medications wisely

The effectiveness of your medication depends in large part on you. When, how and with what you take your pills are important.

Taking your medication correctly

You need to take your pills as prescribed. That may sound obvious, but by some estimates only half the people taking high blood pressure medication do so in correct doses at the right time.

If you take your pills too early, you increase the level of the drug in your blood. This overdose can produce symptoms and side effects such as nausea and diarrhea. If you take your pills too late, drug levels decrease and your blood pressure may increase. And if you stop taking your pills entirely, your blood pressure may rebound to levels higher than before your condition was diagnosed.

It's important to know the names and the doses of all of the medications that you take. To help you remember, keep a list in your purse or wallet and update it when necessary. Here are some tips to help you take your medication properly:

Tie your medication to daily events. If you have a morning medication, put the pills near your breakfast dishes, toothbrush or razor, if this doesn't endanger children or pets. Otherwise, put a sticker near these items to remind you to take your pills.

Set an alarm clock or wristwatch. The alarm will remind you when it's time to take your medication.

Use a plastic pillbox. If you take several drugs, purchase a pillbox with one to three compartments for each day of the week. Load the box once a week to help you keep track of which pills you take and when.

Ask for help from a loved one. Ask him or her to remind you to take your pills, at least until you incorporate the habit into your daily routine.

Take your pills with water. Water helps dissolve the drug. If you generally take your pills with another liquid, check with your doctor or pharmacist to make sure it mixes well with the medication. If you're supposed to take your pills with food, do so. Otherwise the drug may not be absorbed properly into your bloodstream.

Seek good lighting. Don't take your medication in the dark. You might unintentionally take the wrong pill.

Keep the original containers. Occasionally take them to your doctor to make sure you're taking the right drug in the proper dosage.

Note any side effects. Pass this information on to your doctor during your next checkup. Your doctor may want to adjust the dosage or try a different medication. All blood pressure medicine can produce side effects. However, with the right medication, most people experience few problems.

Refill your prescriptions in advance. Plan at least a couple of weeks ahead, in case the unexpected upsets your routine. Snowstorms, the flu and accidents are just a few examples of surprises that can delay your trip to the pharmacy.

Will I ever be able to stop taking medication?

You've taken your medication faithfully, and your blood pressure is within a normal range again. Now you're wondering if you'll one day be able to stop using it. The answer most likely is no.

Some people with high blood pressure that's well controlled are able to reduce the amount of medication they take daily. However, most people continue to take medication the rest of their lives. Blood pressure drugs ensure that your blood pressure stays at a safe level and can lower your risk of complications from uncontrolled hypertension — including stroke, heart attack, heart failure, kidney failure and dementia.

In a few cases, people with stage 1 high blood pressure who have maintained a normal blood pressure for at least a year can discontinue their medication. To do this, your doctor needs to set up a plan for gradually reducing your medication. He or she will also want to see you frequently to make sure your blood pressure doesn't increase again.

To successfully manage your blood pressure without medication, controlling your weight, staying active, eating well and limiting alcohol are essential. Some people who taper off blood pressure drugs eventually need to go back on medication.

If unpleasant side effects are your main reason for wanting to discontinue your medication, a better solution is to work with your doctor to find a way to reduce or eliminate the side effects.

Don't change your dosage. If your blood pressure increases even though you're taking your medication properly, don't increase the dosage on your own. Talk with your doctor first. In addition, don't decrease your dosage without first consulting your doctor.

Preventing interactions

There are more than 80 medications to control high blood pressure. Some can produce dangerous side effects if they're mixed with other prescription drugs, over-the-counter medicines, nutritional and herbal supplements, illicit drugs and even some foods. So it's important that you tell each doctor you see about all of the medications you're taking and to ask about any potentially harmful interactions.

Prescription drugs. Many prescription drugs can interfere with certain blood pressure medications. Again, tell your doctor about every medication you're taking. Some prescription drugs, such as the weight-control medication sibutramine (Meridia), can increase blood pressure.

Anti-inflammatory drugs can interfere with four types of blood pressure medications — diuretics, beta blockers, angiotensin-converting enzyme (ACE) inhibitors, and angiotensin II receptor blockers (ARBs). Another commonly used class of anti-inflammatory medications, called COX-2 inhibitors, is available by prescription. COX-2s include celecoxib (Celebrex), rofecoxib (Vioxx) and valdecoxib (Bextra).

Anti-inflammatory drugs counteract the effects of diuretics by causing your body to retain salt and fluid. They can counteract the effects of beta blockers by preventing the production and release of chemicals that relax your blood vessels. And they can reduce the ability of ACE inhibitors and ARBs to widen your blood vessels.

If you take adult-strength aspirin or another nonsteroidal anti-inflammatory drug (NSAID) or a COX-2 inhibitor regularly, your doctor can adjust the dose of your blood pressure medication to counteract the negative effects of the anti-inflammatory medication. Problems most often develop with intermittent use of anti-inflammatory medications. When taking an NSAID, your blood pressure may rise. Therefore, it's important to tell your doctor about even intermittent anti-inflammatory drug use. Your doctor may want to change your blood pressure medication to a drug less affected by an NSAID. Children-strength aspirin (81 milligram) doesn't affect blood pressure control.

Over-the-counter products. Pain relievers, decongestants and diet pills can pose problems if you're taking blood pressure medication. If you take some of these over-the-counter (OTC) products with certain blood pressure drugs, your blood pressure may increase.

OTC anti-inflammatory medications include the NSAIDs aspirin, ibuprofen (Advil, Motrin, others), ketoprofen (Actron, Orudis KT) and naproxen sodium (Aleve).

Acetaminophen (Tylenol, others) isn't an anti-inflammatory drug, and it doesn't interfere with blood pressure medications.

Use cold and allergy products carefully. Read labels to see if they contain a decongestant such as pseudoephedrine or phenylephrine (used in nasal sprays). Pseudoephedrine and phenylephrine relieve congestion by narrowing blood vessels, minimizing blood flow to an area. This narrowing of blood vessels can increase your blood pressure. Ask your doctor for guidance.

Illicit drugs. Cocaine narrows and inflames your blood vessels and interferes with the effects of blood pressure medications. Street drugs also can cause dangerous drug interactions.

Food. Grapefruit and grapefruit juice can interfere with your liver's ability to remove certain calcium antagonists from your blood. This causes the drug to build up in your body, which can lead to annoying or harmful side effects. If you take the drugs felodipine (Plendil), nifedipine (Adalat, Procardia) or verapamil (Calan SR, Covera-HS, others), don't consume grapefruit or grapefruit juice at all.

Natural licorice, the bittersweet ingredient added to chewing tobacco and licorice cough drops, can increase your blood pressure because it contains glycyrrhizic acid. This chemical makes your kidneys retain salt and fluid. If you take a diuretic to remove excess salt and fluids, avoid natural licorice. Artificially flavored licorice — the kind used in candy — isn't a problem.

Reducing medication costs

Many blood pressure medications are expensive, so taking a drug every day for the rest of your life is a costly prospect — one that's magnified if you take two or more drugs daily. However, there are ways you can reduce your medication costs.

Generic drugs. Once a pharmaceutical company's patent on a drug expires — usually after 17 years — other companies are free to make the drug from the same ingredients. This competition often spurs the original supplier to reduce the price. In addition, the cost of the new generic brands is usually lower. The major reason is that generic manufacturers don't have to recoup costs from years of research and development.

Ask your doctor if it's OK for you to take a generic drug. And don't be surprised if the new pills look different from the original.

Generic drugs are often another shape and color. Because of this, read the label carefully to make sure that the dosage is the same as it was for the original drug.

A generic drug doesn't face the same rigorous testing as a new brand name drug. But the Food and Drug Administration does check to ensure that a generic drug delivers the same amount of active ingredient in the same amount of time as the original brand-name drug. Generic drugs must also meet the same standards of identity, quality and purity as required for brand name products. Still, it's a good idea to monitor your blood pressure more frequently when you first start taking a generic drug.

Splitting pills. Pills generally come in various doses. And many times higher-dose pills cost only a small amount more than lower-dose versions. For example, this means that if you need 50-milligram (mg) tablets, you can buy 100-mg tablets, split them in half and save money.

You can purchase an inexpensive pill splitter at medical supply stores and some pharmacies. It's more convenient and accurate than using a knife and a cutting board.

However, not all pills can be split. For example, this technique doesn't work with capsules containing sustained-release granules. The various ingredients aren't evenly distributed on each side of the capsule.

Nor should you split pills that are coated to keep them from dissolving in your stomach. Cutting negates the coating's effect.

In addition, the medication you take may not come in a larger dose that can be evenly divided. The pills must be cut into equal proportions. And if you're taking several medications or have a condition that makes cutting difficult, pill splitting can become an extra hassle.

Check with your doctor or pharmacist before splitting your pills. Make sure it's safe to do so. Even if you do split pills, follow up with your doctor to make sure your medication is working.

Buying in bulk. In addition to comparison shopping for the best buy among pharmacies, check with discount mail-order pharmacies. Many of these are reputable firms endorsed by respected groups such as the AARP.

Nutritional and herbal supplements

Alternative health products are becoming increasingly popular. But they aren't always effective or safe, and they're less regulated than prescription medications. If you're taking a supplement — or considering it — let your doctor know.

Supplements promoted to lower blood pressure

Coenzyme Q-10	Study results are inconclusive on whether it controls blood pressure.
Cola nut	Has effect of increasing blood pressure.
Fish oil capsules containing omega-3 fatty acids	Capsules are high in fat and calories. May produce gastrointestinal side effects, leave fishy aftertaste. Better to eat fish. Some fish contain levels of mercury that may harm an unborn child's nervous system.
Garlic	Study results are mixed. No conclusive evidence it controls blood pressure.
Ginkgo	No conclusive evidence it controls blood pressure.
Green tea	No conclusive evidence it controls blood pressure.
Potassium, calcium and magnesium	May interfere with other medications. Magnesium supplements may cause diarrhea. Excessive potassium can interfere with heart rhythm.
Vitamin C	No conclusive evidence it controls blood pressure.

Supplements that can increase blood pressure

Ephedra (Ephedrine)	Claims to promote weight loss, provide herbal high. Avoid. Causes a dangerous rise in blood pressure and heart rate and serious complications. This ingredient may also be labeled ma-huang and combined with guavana, a source of caffeine.
Licorice root	Claims to cure ulcers, coughs and colds. Avoid. Can increase blood pressure.
Yohimbe	Claims to increase sexual desire. Avoid. Can increase blood pressure.

Prices at discount suppliers are usually 10 percent to 35 percent lower than you'll find at some pharmacies. The discount is available because the clearinghouse buys and sells in bulk.

A disadvantage of buying in bulk is that if you stockpile too much medication, some of it may expire before you can use it. If your doctor changes your medication, you may also end up with medication you can't use. It's best to buy enough for only 3 to 6 months. If, after receiving the medication, you discover you won't be able to use it all before the expiration date, many companies will exchange the pills.

There's another important disadvantage to buying from mail-order suppliers. You miss having a pharmacist who becomes familiar with your history and all of the medications you're taking. However, if you're diligent about keeping your doctors updated on your medications, discount suppliers can provide a safe and wallet-friendly alternative.

Combination drugs. Some blood pressure medications are used together so often that manufacturers have combined the ingredients into single tablets. These combination tablets are usually less expensive than buying the pills individually. If you take more than one blood pressure medication, ask your doctor if the medications come in combination form.

Assistance programs. Some social service organizations and pharmaceutical companies offer free medication or drugs at greatly reduced prices to people facing financial hardship. Your doctor can help refer you to the appropriate social services or drug manufacturer.

A directory of assistance programs is available from the Pharmaceutical Research and Manufacturers of America (PhRMA), 1100 15th St. N.W., Washington, D.C., 20005, 202-835-3400.

Getting regular follow-up care

If you have stage 1 high blood pressure and no evidence of organ damage, your doctor will want to see you again within 1 to 2 months after you start a treatment program. During that first follow-up visit, your doctor will evaluate your progress, determine whether your blood pressure has decreased, and ask about your efforts on lifestyle modification and any side effects if you're taking medication. If your blood pressure hasn't decreased, your doctor may make some changes in your therapy and possibly change your medication.

If you have stage 2 or 3 high blood pressure and other medical problems that complicate your treatment, you may need to see your doctor every 2 to 4 weeks until you have your blood pressure under control.

Once your blood pressure is well controlled, a visit to your doctor once or twice a year is often all that's needed, unless you have a coexisting medical problem, such as diabetes, high cholesterol, or heart or kidney disease. Then, you'll need to see your doctor more frequently.

Follow-up visits typically involve two blood pressure measurements, a general physical examination and some routine tests. The tests can alert your doctor to possible problems resulting from your medication or to a decline in your heart or kidney function related to your high blood pressure. In addition, follow-up visits are a good time to talk with your doctor about issues related to your medication, weight, diet, activity level or other plans for changing your lifestyle.

Unfortunately, close to half the people with high blood pressure don't see their doctor regularly. This may be another reason why most Americans with hypertension don't control of their condition.

Reaching your goal

If your blood pressure doesn't match the goal set by you and your doctor, you may be tempted to give up. But don't. Instead, ask your doctor why your treatment plan isn't working and make adjustments. Reaching a goal blood pressure level can simply take time.

You can help by:

- Learning all you can about high blood pressure. Because you're reading this book, you're already well on your way.
- Practicing good lifestyle habits, such as controlling your weight, eating well, being physically active and limiting alcohol.
- Remaining patient and optimistic.
- Seeing a high blood pressure specialist, if you're not already doing so.

Your family and friends

Educating your family and friends about high blood pressure also is important to helping you manage your condition. If they don't understand the danger that uncontrolled high blood pressure poses to your health, they may unintentionally work against you. This might include offering you unhealthy food, pestering you about the time you spend on physical activities and even complaining about the high cost of your medicine.

If your family and friends fully understand that your life is at risk if you don't control your blood pressure, they can help make sure you eat well and remind you when it's time to take your medication or to go for your daily walk. In fact, they may even join you. That's why it's important that you ask for and welcome their support.

Wrap-up

Key points to remember:

- Monitoring your blood pressure at home can help you stay in control of your condition. You can purchase blood pressure monitors at medical supply stores and some pharmacies.
- If you take blood pressure medication, it's essential that you take it as directed every day. Pillboxes and daily reminders can help you take your pills correctly.
- Generic drugs, buying in bulk, splitting your pills or purchasing combination drugs may be options for reducing your medication costs. Assistance programs might be available if your financial resources are limited.
- Some over-the-counter pain relievers, decongestants and diet pills, as well as prescription anti-inflammatory drugs, can interfere with some blood pressure medications.
- See your doctor as recommended.

Chapter 11

Medications and how they work

The best and safest way to control your blood pressure is through changes in your lifestyle. Sometimes, though, lifestyle changes can't reduce your blood pressure enough. To reach a desirable blood pressure, you may need the help of medication.

Medication is often necessary if you have severe high blood pressure that needs to be reduced more quickly than lifestyle changes can accomplish, or if you have an accompanying medical condition.

Blood pressure medications, known as antihypertensives, are one of the major success stories in modern medicine. They're quite effective, and most people aren't bothered by their side effects. These drugs can control your high blood pressure and allow you to live normally with your condition. You also benefit by reducing your risk of future health problems.

There are several different classes of blood pressure medication. Each lowers blood pressure in a different manner, and within each class there are drugs with more subtle differences in action. If one medication doesn't decrease your blood pressure to a safe level, your doctor may substitute a different type or add another drug to what you're already taking. A combination of two or more low-dose drugs may lower blood pressure as well as one drug alone at full dose can. In addition, lower doses in drug combinations may produce fewer side effects.

Finding the right medication — or combination of medications — can sometimes take time. Factors to consider include your age and overall health, other medications you already take, how you feel while on the medication, how often you must take it and the cost of the medication. The important thing is that you work with your doctor to develop a treatment plan that works for you. This approach may require patience.

The different types

The major classes of medication used to control high blood pressure include:

- Diuretics
- Beta blockers
- Angiotensin-converting enzyme (ACE) inhibitors
- Angiotensin II receptor blockers
- Calcium antagonists (also known as calcium channel blockers)
- Alpha blockers
- Central-acting agents
- Direct vasodilators

In the following sections, drugs are listed alphabetically with their generic name first. If you have questions about a particular medication, talk with your doctor.

Diuretics

These drugs were first introduced in the 1950s, and they're still one of the most commonly used medications to lower blood pressure. Diuretics have two major advantages. They've proved their effectiveness over the years, most recently in the Antihypertensive and Lipid-Lowering Treatment to Prevent Heart Attack Trial (ALLHAT) published in late 2002. ALLHAT researchers found that among about 33,000 people age 55 and older, diuretics were more effective than either ACE inhibitors or calcium antagonists in controlling high blood pressure and preventing complications from cardiovascular disease. Diuretics are also the least expensive of all the blood pressure drugs.

Commonly referred to as water pills, diuretics reduce the volume of fluid in your body. They cause your kidneys to excrete more sodium in your urine than they would normally. The sodium takes with it water from your blood. This effect means there's a smaller volume of blood pushing through your arteries and, consequently, less pressure on your artery walls.

Diuretics are often the first drug of choice for people with stage 1 high blood pressure. They're highly effective in blacks and older adults, who more frequently are sodium sensitive. In addition, they're commonly used in combination with other medications.

If you take a diuretic, it's important that you also limit sodium and get enough potassium in your diet. This will help the drug work more effectively and with fewer side effects.

Types of diuretics

There are three classes of diuretics. Each works by affecting different parts of your kidneys.

Thiazides. These are some thiazide and thiazide-like diuretics:

- Bendroflumethiazide (Naturetin)
- Chlorothiazide (Diuril)
- Chlorthalidone (Hygroton, Thalitone)
- Hydrochlorothiazide (HydroDiuril, Microzide)
- Indapamide (Lozol)
- Methyclothiazide (Aquatensen, Enduron)
- Metolazone (Mykrox, Zaroxolyn)
- Polythiazide (Renese)

In addition to controlling high blood pressure, thiazide diuretics provide other potential benefits. They've been shown to reduce the risk of stroke, heart attack and heart failure in older adults. They also reduce the amount of calcium in your urine, so less calcium is available for kidney stone formation. Less calcium in your urine results in increased amounts in your blood, which can help reduce your chances of developing osteoporosis.

Loop. These diuretics are more powerful than thiazides, removing a larger percentage of sodium from your kidneys. Your doctor may recommend a loop diuretic if thiazides aren't effective or if you have other conditions that also cause your body to retain fluid.

Loop diuretics include:

- Bumetanide (Bumex)
- Ethacrynic acid (Edecrin)
- Furosemide (Lasix)
- Torsemide (Demadex)

Potassium-sparing. In addition to removing sodium from your blood, diuretics remove potassium. Potassium-sparing diuretics help your body retain needed potassium. These drugs are used mainly in combination with thiazides or loop diuretics because they aren't as powerful as the others. Studies show that when taken with other drugs, the potassium-sparing diuretic spironolactone also reduces deaths from heart failure.

Potassium-sparing diuretics include:

- Amiloride (Midamor)
- Eplerenone (Inspra)*
- Spironolactone (Aldactone)
- Triamterene (Dyrenium)

*Eplerenone (Inspra) is a selective aldosterone antagonist and an improved version of the diuretic spironolactone that appears to have fewer side effects. It was approved by the Food and Drug Administration in late 2002.

Side effects and cautions

The leading side effect associated with diuretics is increased urination. Thiazide and loop diuretics can also cause potassium loss. That's why the two may be used in combination with a potassium-sparing diuretic.

In older adults, thiazide diuretics may cause weakness or dizziness on standing. The drugs can also cause impotence in some men, although this is uncommon. Stopping use of your medication usually causes these problems to disappear. But don't do so without your doctor's advice and guidance. In addition, high doses of thiazide diuretics can slightly increase your blood sugar and total blood cholesterol levels. They also can increase the level of uric acid in your cells. In rare cases, this can lead to development of gout, a joint disorder. Another rare condition, this one called hyponatremia, is characterized by low blood sodium concentrations. It occurs in older adults who are taking thiazide diuretics and who drink too much water. Hyponatremia causes headache and confusion, and can lead to coma.

Loop diuretics sometimes can lead to dehydration. Potassium-sparing diuretics can raise your potassium level too much. If you have impaired kidney function, you shouldn't take a potassium-sparing diuretic because it may lead to excessive potassium levels, which can cause serious heart rhythm irregularities.

Beta blockers

Like diuretics, beta blockers have been used for many years and are often a drug of first choice for reducing blood pressure. Beta blockers work especially well in older adults who have heart disease. However, blacks don't respond as well as whites when taking most types of beta blockers for high blood pressure.

These drugs were originally developed to treat coronary artery disease and were later approved for treatment of high blood pressure after studies found a decrease in blood pressure among people taking them.

Beta blockers lower blood pressure by blocking many of the effects of the hormone epinephrine (ep-ih-NEF-rin), also known as adrenaline (uh-DREN-uh-lin), which causes your heart to beat faster and your blood vessels to constrict. The action of a beta blocker is to make your heart beat more slowly and less forcefully, thus helping to lower your blood pressure. They also slow your kidneys' release of the enzyme renin. Renin is involved in the production of angiotensin (an-je-o-TEN-sin) II, another substance that narrows your blood vessels, increasing your blood pressure.

Beta blockers successfully lower blood pressure in about half the people who try them. They're especially helpful if your high blood pressure is accompanied by certain cardiovascular conditions, such as chest pain (angina), an irregular heart rhythm (arrhythmia), heart failure or a previous heart attack. Beta blockers help control these conditions and reduce your risk of a second heart attack.

Beta blockers may also be used to treat glaucoma, migraines, anxiety, hyperthyroidism and some tremors.

Types of beta blockers

If you have liver or kidney problems, your choice of a beta blocker may be more limited. Some beta blockers are broken down (metabolized) in your liver, others are removed by your kidneys and some by both. If, for example, your kidneys aren't functioning properly, a drug that's normally removed by your kidneys may build up to toxic levels.

Beta blockers also are divided according to whether they affect primarily your heart (cardioselective) or your heart and your blood vessels equally (noncardioselective). Cardioselective types generally produce fewer side effects.

Beta blockers used to treat high blood pressure include:

- Acebutolol (Sectral)
- Atenolol (Tenormin)
- Betaxolol (Kerlone)
- Bisoprolol (Zebeta)
- Carteolol (Cartrol)
- Carvedilol (Coreg)*
- Labetalol (Normodyne, Trandate)*
- Metoprolol (Lopressor, Toprol XL)
- Nadolol (Corgard)
- Penbutolol (Levatol)
- Pindolol
- Propranolol (Inderal)
- Timolol (Blocadren)

*These drugs have the activity of a beta blocker and an alpha blocker.

Side effects and cautions

Beta blockers have more-frequent side effects than other blood pressure medications. However, many people who take the drugs are bothered only minimally, or side effects are reduced over time.

Two of the most notable side effects are fatigue and a reduced capacity for strenuous physical activities. Other side effects may include cold hands, trouble sleeping, impotence, loss of sex drive, a slight increase in your blood triglyceride level, hypoglycemia and a slight decrease in your "good" (high-density lipoprotein, or HDL) blood cholesterol level.

Beta blockers aren't the best choice if you're an active young person or a serious athlete because they can limit your ability to be fully physically active. The drugs also aren't recommended if you have asthma or severe blockage in the conducting system of your heart.

ACE inhibitors

Angiotensin-converting enzyme (ACE) inhibitors are a common choice among doctors for treating high blood pressure. They're effective and produce few side effects. Among blacks, ACE inhibitors are most effective when they're combined with a diuretic.

These drugs work by preventing an enzyme from producing a substance called angiotensin II. Angiotensin II narrows your blood vessels, increasing your blood pressure. It stimulates release of the hormone aldosterone, which increases the retention of salt and water. Limiting action of this enzyme also allows another substance called bradykinin (brad-e-KI-nin) — which keeps your vessels widened — to remain in your blood.

ACE inhibitors provide additional benefits beyond lowering blood pressure. They've been shown to prevent and treat cardiovascular disease, including coronary artery disease, heart failure and stroke. ACE inhibitors also delay progression of kidney disease and protect against diabetes.

ACE inhibitors include:

- Benazepril (Lotensin)
- Captopril (Capoten)
- Enalapril (Vasotec)
- Fosinopril (Monopril)
- Lisinopril (Prinivil, Zestril)
- Moexipril (Univasc)
- Perindopril (Aceon)
- Quinapril (Accupril)
- Ramipril (Altace)
- Trandolapril (Mavik)

Side effects and cautions

ACE inhibitors generally cause few side effects, but some people who take them develop a dry cough. This occurs more commonly in women than in men. In some people, the cough can be persistent and annoying enough to warrant switching to another medication. ACE inhibitors can also elevate your potassium level, which can be dangerous if the level rises too high.

Other possible side effects may include a rash, an altered sense of taste and a reduced appetite. If you have severe kidney disease, an ACE inhibitor should be used with caution because it can contribute to kidney failure. ACE inhibitors aren't recommended if you're pregnant or plan to become pregnant. They can cause serious birth defects to the unborn child. Rarely — but more commonly in blacks and in smokers — the medication may cause swelling. This can be a potentially life-threatening condition when the swelling occurs in the throat, obstructing breathing (angioedema).

Angiotensin II receptor blockers

As their name implies, angiotensin II receptor blockers (ARBs) block the action of angiotensin II. On the other hand, ACE inhibitors block the formation of angiotensin II. Angiotensin II receptor blockers are also different from ACE inhibitors in that they don't increase bradykinin.

These drugs are about equally as effective as ACE inhibitors in treating high blood pressure. And ARBs have been shown to be as effective as ACE inhibitors in treating people with heart failure and more effective in treating kidney failure. They also provide the extra benefit of rarely causing a dry cough. The ARB losartan lowers uric acid concentrations in the blood, which can be important if you're taking a thiazide diuretic or have gout.

Angiotensin II receptor blockers include:

- Candesartan (Atacand)
- Eprosartan (Teveten)
- Irbesartan (Avapro)
- Losartan (Cozaar)
- Olmesartan (Benicar)
- Telmisartan (Micardis)
- Valsartan (Diovan)

Side effects and cautions

Side effects are uncommon, but in some people the drugs can cause dizziness, nasal congestion, back and leg pain, diarrhea, indigestion and insomnia. In rare cases the medication may cause angioedema.

Like ACE inhibitors, these drugs should be taken with caution if you have severe kidney disease, and not at all if you're pregnant or you're contemplating pregnancy.

Calcium antagonists

Calcium antagonists — also called calcium channel blockers — are effective and generally well tolerated. Calcium antagonists work by affecting the muscle cells in the walls of your arteries. These muscle cells contain tiny passages in their membranes called calcium channels. When calcium flows into them, your muscle cells contract and your arteries narrow. Calcium antagonists block these channels — just like plugs in drains — and prevent calcium from getting into your muscle cells. The drugs don't, however, affect calcium used in the building of bone.

Some calcium antagonists have an added benefit of slowing your heart rate, potentially reducing your blood pressure even further. They can also help prevent Raynaud's disease, which affects circulation in the hands and the feet.

Types of calcium antagonists

There are two types of calcium antagonists:

Short-acting. These drugs lower your blood pressure quickly, often in a mere half-hour. But their effects last only a few hours.

Short-acting calcium antagonists aren't recommended for treating chronic high blood pressure because they require that you take them three or four times a day. This generally results in poor control of your blood pressure. Some studies also have linked the drugs to increased risk of heart attack and sudden cardiac death.

Long-acting. These drugs are absorbed into your body more gradually. Although it takes them longer to lower your blood pressure, they control it for a longer period.

Studies that combined data from large randomized trials have found long-acting calcium antagonists aren't as effective as diuretics and beta blockers. Compared with ACE inhibitors, calcium antagonists are less effective in reducing heart attacks and kidney failure, but more effective in reducing stroke. The recent Antihypertensive and Lipid-Lowering Treatment to Prevent Heart Attack Trial (ALLHAT) referred to earlier in this chapter confirmed that diuretics were more effective than calcium antagonists in lowering blood pressure and in preventing heart failure.

Long-acting calcium antagonists used for treating high blood pressure include:

- Amlodipine (Norvasc)
- Diltiazem (Cardizem, Dilacor XR, others)*
- Felodipine (Plendil)
- Isradipine (DynaCirc)
- Nicardipine (Cardene)
- Nifedipine (Adalat, Procardia)
- Nisoldipine (Sular)
- Verapamil (Calan SR, Covera-HS, others)*

*These drugs also slow your heart rate and are useful in treating certain heart arrythmias and angina, and in preventing second heart attacks and migraines.

Side effects and cautions

Possible side effects include constipation, headache, a rapid heartbeat, a rash, swollen feet and lower legs, and swollen gums.

You shouldn't take felodipine (Plendil), nifedipine (Adalat, Procardia), nisoldipine (Sular) and verapamil (Calan SR, Covera-HS, others) with grapefruit or grapefruit juice at all. A substance in the juice seems to reduce your liver's ability to eliminate these calcium antagonists from your body, allowing the drugs to build up and become toxic.

Alpha blockers

Alpha blockers lower your blood pressure by reducing the effect of the hormone norepinephrine (noradrenaline), which stimulates the muscles in the walls of your smaller arteries and veins. As a result, the walls don't narrow (constrict) as much. For older men with prostate problems, alpha blockers also improve urine flow and reduce awakenings at night to go to the bathroom.

Alpha blockers have been used to treat high blood pressure for more than two decades. However, their use is being re-evaluated following the early conclusion in March 2000 of a portion of the ALLHAT study referred to earlier. ALLHAT researchers found that the alpha blocker doxazosin (Cardura) provided less benefit than traditional diuretics, and a higher percentage of people taking doxazosin developed congestive heart failure than did those taking other blood pressure medications. Due to this finding, the NHLBI advises against taking an alpha blocker alone to control high blood pressure. It also recommends that people taking alpha blockers consult their doctors about the benefits and disadvantages of continuing the medication.

Alpha blockers are available in both short-acting and long-acting forms. They include:

- Doxazosin (Cardura), a long-acting drug
- Prazosin (Minipress), a short-acting drug
- Terazosin (Hytrin), a long-acting drug

Side effects and cautions

These drugs are generally well tolerated. However, when you first begin taking the drug or if you're older, it can cause you to feel dizzy or actually faint when you stand up. That's because alpha blockers slow the time it takes your body to respond to the natural change in blood pressure when you move from a sitting or lying position to a standing position. Other possible side effects include headache, a pounding heartbeat, nausea and weakness.

Central-acting agents

Unlike other blood pressure medications that work on your blood vessels, central-acting agents work on your brain. They prevent your brain from sending signals to your nervous system to speed up your heart rate and narrow your blood vessels.

These medications, also called central adrenergic (ad-ren-UR-jik) inhibitors, aren't used as often as they once were because they can produce strong side effects. However, they're still prescribed in certain circumstances. Your doctor may recommend a central-acting agent if you're prone to panic attacks, you have hot flashes, or incidents of low blood sugar, or you're going through alcohol or drug withdrawal. The drugs can help reduce symptoms of these conditions.

One type of central-acting agent, clonidine, is available as a skin patch. This is helpful if you have trouble taking oral medication.

Another type of central-acting agent, methyldopa, is often recommended to pregnant women with high blood pressure who can't take other blood pressure drugs because of risks to themselves and the baby.

Central-acting agents include:

- Clonidine (Catapres)
- Guanabenz (Wytensin)
- Guanadrel (Hylorel)*
- Guanfacine (Tenex)
- Methyldopa (Aldomet)
- Reserpine

*This drug works primarily on the nervous system outside of the brain.

Side effects and cautions

These drugs can produce extreme fatigue, drowsiness, dizziness or sedation. They can also cause impotence, dry mouth, weight gain, impaired thinking and psychological problems, including depression.

Stopping use of some central-acting agents can cause your blood pressure to increase to dangerously high levels very quickly. If you're bothered by side effects and want to quit taking your drug, see your doctor and develop a plan for gradually stopping its use.

Direct vasodilators

These potent medications are used mainly to treat difficult cases of high blood pressure that don't respond well to other medications. They work directly on the muscles in the walls of your arteries, preventing the muscles from tightening and your arteries from narrowing.

Direct vasodilators include:

- Fenoldopam (Corlopam)
- Hydralazine (Apresoline)
- Minoxidil (Loniten)

Side effects and cautions

Common side effects of direct vasodilators include a fast heartbeat, dizziness and retention of water — none of which is very desirable if you have high blood pressure. That's why doctors typically prescribe direct vasodilators with a beta blocker and a diuretic, which can reduce these symptoms. Other side effects may include gastrointestinal problems, dizziness, headache, nasal congestion and swelling of your gums. Taking Minoxidil may result in excessive hair growth. Hydralazine taken in large doses can increase your risk of lupus, a connective tissue disease.

Emergency medications

If your blood pressure reaches a dangerously high level, it may be necessary to reduce it rapidly to avoid serious damage to your organs, and even death. These risks include heart attack, heart failure, stroke, sudden blindness or a rupture in the wall of your aorta.

During blood pressure emergencies, doctors inject a blood pressure lowering medication directly into your bloodstream. The goal is to lower your blood pressure by 25 percent within several minutes to 2 hours. Reducing your blood pressure too fast can cause other serious, even fatal, conditions. Once your blood pressure is reduced 25 percent, then the goal is to lower your blood pressure to near 160/100 millimeters of mercury (mm Hg) within 6 hours.

Injectable medications used in hypertensive emergencies include:

- Vasodilators, such as fenoldopam, nicardipine hydrochloride, nitroglycerin, sodium nitroprusside and hydralazine
- Alpha and beta blockers, such as phentolamine, esmolol and labetalol
- The ACE inhibitor enalaprilat

Combination drug therapy

Approximately half the people with stage 1 or 2 high blood pressure can control their blood pressure with just one drug. If one drug isn't effective, your doctor may increase the dosage, provided you aren't experiencing significant side effects. Other options are to try a different drug or add another drug to the one you're already taking. Generally, if a diuretic isn't the first drug prescribed, it may be the second.

By using a combination of two or more drugs, doctors can increase from 50 percent to 80 percent the number of people who

Working in combination

It's common for two drugs to be mixed together into the same tablet or capsule. Some examples of high blood pressure medications in which two drugs are combined into one are listed here.

Combinations of a beta blocker and a diuretic:

- Nadolol and bendroflumethiazide (Corzide)
- Atenolol and chlorthalidone (Tenoretic)
- Bisoprolol and hydrochlorothiazide (Ziac)
- Propranolol and hydrochlorothiazide (Inderide LA)
- Metoprolol and hydrochlorothiazide (Lopressor HCT)

Combinations of an angiotensin-converting enzyme (ACE) inhibitor and a diuretic:

- Benazepril and hydrochlorothiazide (Lotensin HCT)
- Captopril and hydrochlorothiazide (Capozide)
- Enalapril and hydrochlorothiazide
- Lisinopril and hydrochlorothiazide (Prinzide, Zestoretic)

Combinations of an angiotensin II receptor antagonist and a diuretic:

- Losartan potassium and hydrochlorothiazide (Hyzaar)
- Valsartan and hydrochlorothiazide (Diovan HCT)

Combinations of two diuretics:

- Amiloride and hydrochlorothiazide (Moduretic)
- Spironolactone and hydrochlorothiazide (Aldactazide)
- Triamterene and hydrochlorothiazide (Dyazide, Maxzide)

Combinations of a calcium antagonist and an ACE inhibitor:

- Amlodipine and benazepril (Lotrel)
- Trandolapril and verapamil (Tarka)
- Enalapril and felodipine (Lexxel)

respond positively to high blood pressure medication. Your doctor looks for medications that enhance each other's effectiveness or reduce each other's side effects. If you have another medical condition and your blood pressure goal is lower than 130/80 mm Hg, you may need three or more classes of medications. For more on special concerns and conditions, see Chapter 12.

Finding the right medication

Almost all people taking blood pressure medication are eventually able to come up with a drug regimen that allows them to feel good and be fully active, and that also produces few, if any, side effects. In addition to the effectiveness of a drug, your doctor will consider:

Your tolerance to the drug. If taking a certain medication produces side effects that are unpleasant to live with, such as impotence or headaches, then it's probably not the best drug for you. In fact, the medication's side effects may seem worse to live with than your high blood pressure, which produces no apparent symptoms. But don't stop taking the medication on your own. Talk to your doctor.

Your compliance with the prescription. If a certain medication is complicated to take and you have a busy schedule, you may forget to take it. Because it's vital that you take your medication properly, the medication your doctor prescribes should fit your lifestyle. In most cases, it's possible to be taking just one medication once daily.

Your ability to pay for the medication. A drug doesn't do you any good if you can't take it correctly because you can't afford it. Let your doctor know if you can't afford your medication.

Gene research

Beyond your risk of disease, your genes affect how you respond to medication, including drug therapy for high blood pressure. If gene

On the horizon

Dual metalloprotease inhibitors block a substance that narrows your arteries and increase another that opens them wider. The first drug in this class — omapatrilat (Vanlev) — has been shown to be more effective than a commonly used angiotensin-converting enzyme (ACE) inhibitor. However, it has caused higher rates of angioedema than has the ACE inhibitor and is receiving further study.

For information about new drugs or to learn more about existing medications, visit our Web site at *www.MayoClinic.com.*

research is successful, it may lead not only to the development of new drugs, but also to the better selection of drugs. By knowing your genetic makeup, your doctor may then be able to determine the type of medication that's most likely to be effective and beneficial for you.

For example, a team of researchers, including doctors at Mayo Clinic, identified a gene (GNB3) that may play a role in how people respond to certain diuretics. They found that people with one variation of the gene responded better to the medication and had lower blood pressures than did people with another variation of the gene.

Wrap-up

Key points to remember:

- You may need medication if lifestyle changes aren't effective, you have severe high blood pressure or you have another medical condition that could benefit from drug use.
- Half the people with high blood pressure needing medication can control their blood pressure with just one drug. Others need a combination of two or three drugs.
- A diuretic, beta blocker or angiotensin-converting enzyme (ACE) inhibitor is often prescribed for uncomplicated high blood pressure because of their successful track records.
- Most people taking blood pressure medication are bothered only minimally by side effects.
- Finding the right drug or combination of drugs to control your blood pressure may require time and patience.

Chapter 12

Special concerns and conditions

High blood pressure most often develops between the ages of 30 and 60, but it has no boundaries. It can affect anyone at any time. Your blood pressure is influenced by your sex, race and certain medical conditions. When determining the best way to treat or prevent high blood pressure, all of these factors must be considered.

This chapter looks at factors unique to women and children, management of high blood pressure among specific populations and groups, treatment of difficult-to-control high blood pressure, and what to do in a hypertensive emergency.

Issues for women

Until recently, most studies on the development and the treatment of high blood pressure primarily involved men. Yet, approximately 60 percent of all people diagnosed with high blood pressure are women.

As it becomes apparent that women may respond differently to medication and that they often develop the disease for different reasons and at different times in their lives, more studies are now focusing on issues that affect women.

Oral contraceptives

Oral contraceptives — the pill — are a common form of birth control. They contain small amounts of the hormones estrogen and progestin that prevent pregnancy.

When oral contraceptives first came on the market decades ago, they contained much larger doses of estrogen and progestin than they do now. Back then, about 5 percent of all women who took oral contraceptives developed high blood pressure. Today, the hormone dose in oral contraceptives is about 80 percent less than that in earlier versions, and high blood pressure from oral contraceptives is uncommon. The drugs may cause your systolic blood pressure to increase slightly.

If you're a woman whose blood pressure does increase significantly with use of an oral contraceptive, your doctor may recommend that you stop taking the pill. Within a few months, your blood pressure should return to normal. If alternative birth control isn't possible and you want to continue taking the pill, you'll need to take steps to lower your blood pressure through lifestyle changes and possibly medication.

A newer contraceptive that combines drospirenone and ethinyl estradiol (Yasmin) contains a new kind of synthetic progestin. This drug can cause you to retain potassium and could lead to abnormally high levels of potassium in your blood if you're also taking a potassium-sparing diuretic or other medication to manage your high blood pressure.

Pregnancy

It's quite possible for women with high blood pressure to have a normal pregnancy and childbirth. However, if you have high blood pressure, you have a greater risk of complications during your pregnancy, which can affect both you and your unborn child.

Your doctor will want to monitor your pregnancy and your blood pressure closely, especially during the last 3 months (third trimester), when complications are most likely to occur.

Uncommon, but possible, complications for the mother include heart failure, seizures, a decline in kidney or liver function, vision changes, and bleeding. Possible complications for the fetus include impaired growth, greater risk of separation of the placenta from the uterine wall, and greater risk of reduced oxygen during labor.

Talk with your doctor about possible health risks before becoming pregnant. You may change your medication because some blood pressure drugs shouldn't be taken during pregnancy. Also, inform your doctor as soon as you become pregnant.

If you see a different doctor during your pregnancy, make sure to mention during your first visit that you have high blood pressure. Because blood pressure normally decreases during the early and middle stages of pregnancy, a doctor who's unfamiliar with your medical history may not realize you have high blood pressure.

If you have stage 2 or stage 3 high blood pressure, your doctor will likely recommend that you continue to take your medication while you're pregnant. The benefit you receive from the medication usually outweighs the risk of side effects to your developing baby.

If you have stage 1 high blood pressure, discuss with your doctor the benefits and disadvantages of taking medication. For high-normal high blood pressure, it's not clear that the benefits of continuing your medication outweigh the possible risks to your baby.

For women who need to take high blood pressure medication during pregnancy, the central-acting drug methyldopa (meth-ul-DO-puh) is sometimes used. Beta blockers also may be prescribed in certain situations. Angiotensin-converting enzyme (ACE) inhibitors and angiotensin II receptor blockers (ARBs) shouldn't be taken during pregnancy because they can potentially slow growth of the fetus, cause birth defects and possibly be fatal to the fetus.

Pregnancy-induced high blood pressure. A small percentage of women develop high blood pressure during their pregnancy. This condition is sometimes referred to as gestational hypertension. It most often happens during the later stages of pregnancy, and in most cases the increase is mild. Once the pregnancy is complete, blood pressure returns to normal.

If you develop pregnancy-induced high blood pressure — especially if you have stage 1 high blood pressure — medication generally isn't necessary. But you may need to limit sodium and follow a diet that emphasizes grains, fruits, vegetables and low-fat dairy products — foods that help control high blood pressure.

Only if your blood pressure increases a significant amount, putting your health or your baby's health in jeopardy, is medication recommended.

In most cases, pregnancy-induced high blood pressure is a sign of one of two things. It's an early indicator that you're likely to develop high blood pressure later in life, or it's an early warning of a condition called preeclampsia.

Preeclampsia. In the past 10 years, the number of cases of preeclampsia (pre-e-KLAMP-se-uh) in the United States has increased by nearly one-third. Preeclampsia is a condition that occurs in approximately 7 percent of pregnant women. It's characterized by a significant increase in blood pressure and excess protein in the urine. It typically develops after the 20th week of pregnancy. Left untreated, preeclampsia can lead to serious, even deadly, complications.

The exact cause of preeclampsia is unknown. Certain factors, though, can increase your risk of preeclampsia. They include:

- Pre-existing chronic high blood pressure
- A first pregnancy
- A family history of preeclampsia
- Carrying multiple fetuses
- Diabetes
- Kidney problems before pregnancy
- Pregnancy at either end of childbearing years — early teens or late 30s into your 40s

Two factors that may contribute to the increase in preeclampsia are more women having children later in life and more multiple births.

Women who develop preeclampsia often have no symptoms at first. By the time they do appear, the condition is often advanced. In addition to having increased protein in your urine, you may experience sudden weight gain of more than 2 pounds (0.9 kilogram) in a week or 6 pounds (2.7 kilograms) in a month. Other signs and symptoms may include headache, vision problems and pain in your upper abdomen.

Your blood pressure and urine generally will be checked routinely during your pregnancy. Your doctor also may perform blood tests to check your blood platelet count and to see how well your liver and kidneys are functioning. A low-blood-platelet level and increased liver enzyme values indicate a severe form of preeclampsia called HELLP (hemolysis, elevated liver enzymes, low platelet count) syndrome.

Severe preeclampsia requires you to stay in the hospital. Your health and that of your baby's are continuously monitored. You may be given medication to help control your blood pressure and help prevent seizures. If tests indicate that your health or your baby's health may be at significant risk, early delivery of your baby may be necessary. Labor may be induced or a Caesarean section performed.

Mild preeclampsia often can be managed at home with bed rest. You'll be asked to lie on your left side to allow blood to flow more freely to the placenta. Your doctor will want to see you frequently to check your blood pressure and urine, do blood tests, and check the status of the baby. You also may need to check your blood pressure on a regular basis at home. To prevent the condition from worsening, your doctor may recommend delivery at 38 weeks instead of waiting until labor begins normally.

After delivery, your blood pressure should return to normal within several days to several weeks. If your blood pressure is still at stage 2 or stage 3 when you leave the hospital you may need to take blood pressure medication. Most women are able to taper off the medication after a few months.

Eclampsia. Eclampsia is a life-threatening condition that can develop when symptoms of preeclampsia aren't controlled. The incidence of eclampsia is about 1 in 1,500 pregnancies.

Signs and symptoms of eclampsia include:

- Pain in the upper-right side of your abdomen
- Severe headache and vision problems, including seeing flashing lights
- Convulsions
- Unconsciousness

Eclampsia can permanently damage your brain, liver or kidneys, and it can be fatal for both you and your unborn child. Emergency delivery of the baby is necessary.

Hormone replacement therapy

Unlike oral contraceptives — in which the hormones estrogen and progestin may slightly increase your blood pressure — in hormone replacement therapy (HRT) these hormones don't raise blood pressure. According to some studies, HRT may even slightly reduce blood pressure.

The difference in effect is related mainly to the level of estrogen. HRT contains considerably lower doses of estrogen than do oral contraceptives. Another reason may be that HRT contains different types of progestin or no progestin at all.

HRT is often prescribed to women for a limited time after menopause to reduce postmenopausal symptoms, such as hot flashes and vaginal dryness. It's also prescribed to reduce the risk of fractures due to osteoporosis. Until recently, it was prescribed to reduce the risk of cardiovascular disease and some forms of cancer. But two studies found that HRT offered no benefit in reducing heart attacks in women already diagnosed with cardiovascular disease, and that it slightly increased the risk of some forms of cancer. Talk with your doctor about whether taking HRT is appropriate for you.

High blood pressure in children

Infants are born with a low blood pressure that increases quickly during the first month of life. During childhood, your blood pressure continues to slowly increase until you reach your teens, when it reaches a level similar to that in an adult.

Blood pressure generally isn't measured routinely in infants and toddlers because it's difficult to get an accurate reading. However, young children can develop high blood pressure, and just as with adults, it may not always be accompanied by symptoms. It may not be until such problems occur as unexplained irritability, vomiting or failure to grow properly — or in extreme cases seizures or heart failure — that high blood pressure may be suspected.

When your child reaches age 3, it's appropriate to have his or her blood pressure checked at every well-child visit. To determine whether your child's blood pressure is truly elevated, blood pressure is rated on a percentile basis, taking into account his or her age and height. At any age, taller children tend to have higher blood pressures than do children who are shorter or of average height. A child with a blood pressure reading in the 5-percent range above the 95th percentile is considered to have high blood pressure.

Between 1 percent and 3 percent of children in the United States have persistent high blood pressure. As an increasing number of children become less physically active and more obese, more run the risk of developing high blood pressure in their teens.

More often than in adults, high blood pressure in children is associated with a clearly defined cause. Those causes may include narrowing of a kidney artery, kidney failure and hormonal abnormalities. Head trauma, brain infections and tumors also can cause high blood pressure. Coarctation of the aorta, a congenital problem that causes high blood pressure in the upper part of the body, may not be detected until later in life.

Because there may be a clear cause, your doctor will likely perform several tests to find the reason for your child's increased blood pressure. If all test results are normal and all other possible causes are eliminated, then the child is considered to have essential hypertension. The condition may be related to lifestyle factors such as obesity, poor diet and lack of exercise. If more than one child in a family has high blood pressure, there may be a genetic link.

For children with essential hypertension, lifestyle changes are a common treatment. It can be hard for youngsters to stick to a healthy diet and regular exercise plan, especially for teenagers who want to control their own lifestyle choices. Making these goals family priorities reinforces the importance of these changes to your child's and your family's future health. High blood pressure in children that's ignored or not controlled can lead to the same kinds of problems as experienced by adults with the condition, including damage to organs such as the heart, brain, eyes and kidneys.

Your doctor may prescribe medication if your child's blood pressure is quite high or if lifestyle changes alone aren't working. The same medications used to control high blood pressure in adults are used for children, only in smaller doses. For more on medications, see Chapter 11. Some clearly identifiable causes may be remedied with surgery.

High blood pressure in older adults

There was a time when high blood pressure in older adults was ignored because it wasn't thought to be a problem. However, studies have shown that no matter what your age, controlling high blood pressure can reduce your risk of stroke, heart attack, heart failure and progressive kidney failure — and add quality years to your life. Controlling high blood pressure may also prevent memory loss and dementia.

With age, your diastolic blood pressure decreases slightly, but your systolic blood pressure often increases. That's because your blood vessels become more rigid as you get older, causing your heart to work harder to pump blood throughout your body. The vessels simply can't stretch to accommodate the same amount of blood, so the pressure on your artery walls becomes greater.

If your systolic pressure increases to 140 millimeters of mercury (mm Hg) or greater while your diastolic measurement stays normal (less than 90 mm Hg), then you may have a condition called isolated systolic hypertension (ISH). About half the older adults with high blood pressure have this condition.

Doctors were once reluctant to treat ISH because they thought it was a normal result of aging. However, a 5-year study showed that treating this form of high blood pressure in Americans could prevent as many as 24,000 strokes and 44,000 severe cardiovascular problems, including heart attack, each year. Similar studies in Europe and China also show positive results.

Losing weight if you're overweight and walking daily to stay active can help reduce your blood pressure. Because you may become more sodium sensitive with age, limiting sodium to less than 2,400 milligrams daily also may help. In a study involving 681 men and women ages 60 to 80 who initially were taking antihypertensive medication, it was found that reducing sodium intake and losing weight enabled a significant number to remain off medication for 4 years.

If you do need medication in addition to lifestyle changes to lower your blood pressure, the choice of class of drug will depend on other illnesses and risk factors that you have.

Pulse pressure

Pulse pressure is the difference between your systolic and diastolic pressure readings. For example, if your systolic pressure is 120 millimeters of mercury (mm Hg) and your diastolic is 80 mm Hg, your pulse pressure is 40. High pulse pressure — more than 50 mm Hg — may be a sign of isolated systolic hypertension (ISH) in which systolic pressure is quite high, but diastolic remains normal. A high pulse pressure in older adults increases the risk of cardiovascular disease and stroke. Pulse pressure and the accompanying risks are often reduced with a reduction in systolic pressure.

High blood pressure and ethnic groups

As far back as 1932, researchers noted a difference in blood pressures between whites and blacks of African-American descent living in New Orleans. Blood pressures among 6,000 black males were 7 mm Hg higher than among a group of 8,000 white males.

If you're black, you're twice as likely to develop high blood pressure than if you're white. You're also more likely to be overweight, have diabetes, develop insulin resistance syndrome, or to develop serious complications or to die of a stroke, heart attack or kidney failure related to your high blood pressure. Less access to medical care is one factor. However, genetic differences are primarily why more blacks than whites have high blood pressure.

The good news is that with proper medical care, strokes, heart attacks and progressive kidney failure from high blood pressure can be reduced equally as well in blacks as in whites. In addition, black participants in the DASH-Sodium dietary study experienced the greatest reduction in blood pressure. Blacks also benefit more than whites from increasing their potassium intake.

The prevalence of high blood pressure among some populations of American Indians is higher than in whites. Among Hispanics, Asian-Americans and Pacific Islanders, the incidence of high blood pressure is slightly lower than in whites.

High blood pressure and other conditions

Often, high blood pressure is accompanied by other medical conditions that make it more difficult to treat and control. If you have another chronic illness in addition to high blood pressure, it's especially important that you see your doctor regularly.

Cardiovascular problems

Cardiovascular conditions that often coexist with high blood pressure include:

Arrhythmia. High blood pressure can cause your heart to beat in an irregular rhythm. You're at greater risk of developing this condition if your blood contains low levels of potassium or magnesium. This sometimes happens when you're taking a diuretic.

To control or prevent arrhythmia, with your doctor's consent, eat plenty of foods containing potassium and magnesium. If this doesn't help, your doctor may recommend that you take supplements to keep your potassium and magnesium levels normal. In addition, taking a fish oil supplement also may help. Fish oil, which is high in omega-3 fatty acids, has been shown to lower the risk of sudden death due to arrhythmia.

Arteriosclerosis and atherosclerosis. If you have one or both of these conditions, which cause your arteries to become stiff or narrowed, your doctor may prescribe a low-dose diuretic or a beta blocker to reduce the volume or intensity of blood flowing through your arteries. ACE inhibitors and ARBs also may help in reversing the stiffness in your blood vessels.

Coronary artery disease. If you have high blood pressure, there's a 50-percent chance that the major arteries serving your heart (coronary arteries) are damaged. Damage to these arteries increases your risk of a heart attack.

Beta blockers, ACE inhibitors and ARBs are often used to treat people with high blood pressure and coronary artery disease because in addition to lowering blood pressure, they reduce the risk of a heart attack and heart failure. A calcium antagonist may be prescribed to relieve angina and, in some cases, reduce the risk of a second heart attack. A low-dose regimen of aspirin (81 milligrams) for people with controlled high blood pressure can help reduce the risk of cardiovascular problems and the recurrence of heart attack and stroke.

Heart failure. If you have heart failure, you want to keep your blood pressure below 130/85 mm Hg. Heart failure is usually the result of an enlarged, weakened heart, which has a hard time pumping enough blood to meet your body's needs. In some cases, this can cause fluid to build up in your lungs or your feet and legs. For this reason, your doctor will aim for a lower blood pressure so that your heart won't have to work as hard.

An ACE inhibitor and diuretics may be prescribed if you have heart failure in addition to high blood pressure. ACE inhibitors reduce blood pressure by dilating your blood vessels, without interfering with your heart's pumping action. Diuretics reduce fluid buildup. The diuretic spironolactone has been shown to have lifesaving benefits in people with heart failure. In most cases a beta blocker also may be appropriate. If you don't tolerate ACE inhibitors, an ARB may be prescribed instead. Depending on your circumstances, you may chose to see a heart failure specialist because treatment programs are complex and a heart transplant may need to be considered.

Stroke and transient ischemic attack. High blood pressure increases your risk of stroke and transient ischemic attack (TIA). If you're older than 55 and have a high pulse pressure (See "Pulse pressure" on page 181), you may be at an even greater risk. Being black or Asian-American also increases your risk.

Thrombolytic therapy can help reduce the effects of an ischemic stroke if it's given within the first several hours after the onset of symptoms. If you think that you're having a stroke, seek emergency medical treatment immediately.

If you've had a stroke, your doctor may start you on a diuretic and a beta blocker to help reduce your risk of a second stroke. ACE inhibitors, ARBs and calcium antagonists also may be prescribed. Using these drugs to lower blood pressure can reduce the risk of another stroke even if you've never had high blood pressure. One study found that ACE inhibitors were especially effective at reducing stroke risk, particularly in people with stroke risk factors.

Diabetes

High blood pressure is nearly twice as common in people with diabetes. If you're black, your chances of having both diabetes and high blood pressure are double that of a white person. If you're Hispanic, that chance increases to three times. Although Hispanics have about the same risk of high blood pressure as whites, their risk of diabetes is much higher.

Whatever your ethnic group, having both diabetes and high blood pressure is serious. Between 35 percent and 75 percent of all complications associated with diabetes can be attributed to having high blood pressure. High blood pressure also increases your chances for death from diabetes.

If you have diabetes and high blood pressure, you want to reduce your blood pressure to 130/80 mm Hg or lower. If you have kidney disease, your doctor may recommend an even lower blood pressure goal.

To reduce your risk of serious complications from diabetes and high blood pressure, eat a healthy diet, get regular physical activity, limit your use of alcohol, and if you smoke or chew tobacco, stop doing so. A combination of high blood pressure, diabetes and tobacco use puts you at very high risk of a heart attack.

If you need to take blood pressure medication, ACE inhibitors or ARBs are prescribed most often. They help protect your kidneys, which are at a high risk of damage from both diseases. These drugs also have relatively few side effects. Diuretics, beta blockers, calcium antagonists or alpha blockers also may be used to achieve lower blood pressure goals and to prolong life. Often, multiple-drug therapy is needed to get to your goal pressure.

High cholesterol

Eighty percent of people with high blood pressure also have high cholesterol. Because increases in cholesterol and blood pressure raise your risk of a heart attack and stroke, it's important to lower your cholesterol levels as well as your blood pressure.

The same lifestyle changes that lower blood pressure can also help to lower cholesterol levels. However, many people with high cholesterol also need a cholesterol-lowering medication.

As for blood pressure medications, don't take high doses of thiazide and loop diuretics if you also have high cholesterol. They can increase your cholesterol level and your triglycerides, another type of blood fat. Low doses of these drugs, though, don't produce these effects. Beta blockers also may slightly raise your cholesterol. However, should you need to take high doses of a beta blocker, diet and cholesterol medication can help counteract the cholesterol increase. It's also important to remember to avoid eating grapefruit or drinking grapefruit juice if you're taking a statin to lower cholesterol. That's because an interaction between grapefruit juice and the drug can lead to unhealthy levels of the statin in your blood.

Medications most often recommended if you have high blood pressure and high cholesterol are ACE inhibitors, ARBs, calcium antagonists, alpha blockers, central-acting agents and low-dose diuretics.

Insulin resistance syndrome, or metabolic syndrome

The key signs of insulin resistance syndrome (formerly known as syndrome X), also called metabolic syndrome, are obesity, high blood pressure, high triglycerides and low levels of high-density lipoprotein (HDL), or "good" cholesterol. It affects one in three American adults and is more common among blacks. It occurs when your cells become increasingly resistant to insulin and, as a result, your body is less able to process glucose. Your pancreas may compensate by producing more insulin, but over time it's no longer able to overcome the resistance. Glucose accumulates in your body, leading to type 2 diabetes (formerly called adult-onset or noninsulin-dependent diabetes). Insulin resistance syndrome can also lead to high blood pressure when excessive insulin in your system interferes with your kidneys' ability to handle salt, which can lead to fluid retention. Risk of insulin resistance may be partly inherited, but being overweight and inactive — factors over which you have control — also are contributors.

Kidney disease

High blood pressure can lead to progressive renal failure, a condition in which your kidneys no longer function. In this end stage, life is sustained with dialysis or a kidney transplant. If you have kidney disease, you need medications and lifestyle changes to prevent further damage to your kidneys as a result of your high blood pressure.

Kidney failure is especially a concern if you're black. Blacks are nearly four times more likely than are whites to have end-stage renal disease.

Your goal should be to reduce your blood pressure to below 130/80 mm Hg, or lower if you have severe kidney disease. Once your blood pressure is decreased, decline in kidney function slows. If you have advanced renal failure, you'll likely have special dietary needs which are best discussed with a dietitian.

Multiple drugs are necessary in order to reach a blood pressure goal. ACE inhibitors and ARBs are often the best medications for preventing further damage to your kidneys. However, they need to be used with caution. ACE inhibitors and ARBs are commonly combined with a diuretic, especially when treating kidney failure in blacks.

Sexual dysfunction

The prevalence of sexual dysfunction increases with age in both men and women. Some evidence indicates that erectile dysfunction (ED) is higher in men with untreated high blood pressure than in those who take medication. Diuretics may be associated with ED. Beta blockers haven't been associated with ED any more than other antihypertensive drugs. Before starting a high blood pressure medication, discuss your current sexual function with your doctor and report any changes after beginning the medication. Another medication may be available that doesn't interfere with your sexual function. If this approach fails, sildenafil (Viagra) is generally an acceptable treatment for men with ED and high blood pressure. Ask your doctor if it's appropriate for you.

Difficult-to-control high blood pressure

What if you've been following your doctor's orders and taking your medication, but you still aren't able to lower your blood pressure?

It could be you're among 5 percent to 10 percent of people with hypertension whose blood pressure is resistant, or refractory, which means it doesn't fully respond to treatment. Resistant high blood pressure is defined as blood pressure that can't be brought below 140/90 mm Hg using a combination of three different types of medication, including a diuretic.

Are your readings misleading?

In rare cases, resistant high blood pressure may be the result of a mistake in your diagnosis. Two conditions can make your blood pressure appear higher than it actually is. They are:

- Pseudohypertension
- White-coat hypertension

See Chapter 3 for more on these conditions.

It's rare for medication not to lower high blood pressure to the goal. Often, it just takes time and experimentation with different drugs to find the combination of drugs that works best. Try to be patient.

If your medication isn't working, many times the first step is to try a different type of drug. Some medications work better for some people than for others. The next step may be to add another medication to the one you're already taking, perhaps even a third or — if you have diabetes or kidney failure and have lower blood pressure goals — even a fourth drug. Medications often have more powerful effects on your blood pressure when working together than when working alone. Rarely does anyone start out taking three different medications, but sometimes this approach may be necessary.

Often, resistant high blood pressure stems from not making necessary changes in your lifestyle. If your blood pressure isn't responding to drug therapy, ask yourself the following questions:

- *Have I been taking my medication exactly as prescribed?* You need to take your medication as your doctor ordered, or it may not work. If you think the pills cost too much or you find the regimen too hard to follow, talk to your doctor. Less expensive medications that you take only once a day can often be found. It's also important that you tell your doctor about all of the drugs you take, including over-the-counter products. They could be interfering with your blood pressure medication.
- *Have I cut down on sodium?* Remember, this doesn't mean table salt alone. Even if you aren't salting your foods, you may be

eating processed foods with too much sodium. Read package labels to determine how much sodium is contained in a serving.

- *Am I drinking too much alcohol?* Alcohol can keep your blood pressure elevated, especially if you consume large amounts during short intervals. Your medication may not be enough to overcome the effects of alcohol, and the alcohol may interfere with the normal action of the drug.
- *Have I seriously tried to quit smoking?* Like alcohol, tobacco can keep your blood pressure increased if you smoke or chew frequently.
- *Have I gained weight?* Generally, losing weight decreases your blood pressure. Weight gain — as few as 10 pounds — can increase it and make it harder to control.
- *Have I been sleeping well?* A condition called sleep apnea can increase your blood pressure. It occurs most frequently in older adults. People with sleep apnea stop breathing for short periods during the night. This stresses the heart and can increase blood pressure. Relieving the condition can reduce your blood pressure.

If you, along with your doctor, have exhausted these possibilities, you have a couple of options. To begin with, you may need to consider stepping up positive changes to your lifestyle. If you can walk another block, lose 1 more pound or make more improvements in your diet, your high blood pressure may become less resistant to treatment.

Your other options include adding a fourth drug to your daily regimen or increasing the dosage of your current medication. The danger with each is an increased risk of side effects from the medication. If you aren't already seeing a high blood pressure specialist, ask your doctor for a referral.

High blood pressure emergencies

Throughout this book, you've read how uncontrolled high blood pressure can erode your health by wearing on your body and gradually damaging your organs. Sometimes, though, high blood pressure can suddenly become life-threatening, requiring immediate care. When this happens, it's a hypertensive emergency.

Emergency warning signs

In addition to dangerously high blood pressure, signs and symptoms that often signal a hypertensive emergency include:

- A severe headache, accompanied by confusion and blurred vision
- Severe chest pain
- Marked shortness of breath
- Nausea and vomiting
- Seizures
- Unresponsiveness

Don't drink or eat anything and, if you can, lie down until emergency help arrives or you get to a hospital.

Hypertensive emergencies are rare. They occur when your blood pressure increases to a dangerously high level and is accompanied by other serious symptoms. Generally, a reading of 180/110 mm Hg or greater is considered dangerously high. However, if you have another medical condition, lower elevations in your blood pressure also can trigger a hypertensive emergency. The danger level in children is lower, depending on age and height.

Causes include:

- Forgetting to take your blood pressure medication
- Acute stroke
- Acute heart attack
- Heart failure
- Kidney failure
- Rupture of your aorta
- Interaction between blood pressure medication and another drug
- Postoperative complications
- Eclampsia

To prevent damage to your organs, your blood pressure needs to be lowered promptly but gradually. Lowering it too fast can interfere with normal blood flow, possibly resulting in too little blood to your heart, brain and other organs.

Urgency vs. emergency

If at least three blood pressure measurements taken a few minutes apart produce readings of 180/110 mm Hg or higher but you aren't experiencing any other signs and symptoms, contact your doctor or another health care professional at your doctor's office right away. If that isn't possible, go to a hospital near you. Left untreated for more than a few hours, pressures this high could possibly lead to a medical emergency.

Wrap-up

Key points to remember:

- Oral contraceptives rarely cause or worsen high blood pressure.
- High blood pressure during pregnancy must be monitored closely. It can be a sign of a condition called preeclampsia. Left untreated, preeclampsia can lead to life-threatening eclampsia.
- High blood pressure in children is uncommon. It may be a sign of another health problem.
- There are benefits to treating high blood pressure at any age.
- Blacks have twice the incidence of high blood pressure and more complications from it. Some American Indian populations also have higher rates of high blood pressure.
- High blood pressure associated with diabetes, high cholesterol, cardiovascular disease, stroke or kidney disease needs aggressive treatment.
- Dangerously high blood pressure accompanied by other symptoms requires immediate treatment.

Menus with DASH

The pages that follow include a week of menus developed by Mayo Clinic dietitians, based on the recommendations of the Dietary Approaches to Stop Hypertension (DASH) eating plan.

The menus emphasize grains, vegetables, fruits and low-fat dairy products. This variety helps provide plentiful amounts of the minerals potassium, calcium and magnesium, which help promote healthy blood pressure levels. Each day's menu is based on a diet of 2,000 calories, with no more than 30 percent of calories coming from fat. See "Calculating calories" on page 68 to determine your requirements. A registered dietitian can help you adjust the menus to meet your calorie level. Sodium is limited to less than 2,400 milligrams a day, with occasional suggestions on how to reduce sodium even further.

Accompanying each of the menus is the recipe for the dinner entree. The recipes use commonly available ingredients and are designed with an eye toward ease of preparation.

Use these menus as a guide to adopting a more nutritiously balanced diet. Feel free to make substitutions or adjustments to the menus to suit your tastes. If, for example, you don't care for peaches, you can substitute the peach in the Day 1 menu with another fruit, such as an apple or a serving of strawberries. The idea is to enjoy a variety of foods in your daily diet.

Day 1

Breakfast

2 oatmeal pancakes, topped with ½ cup (4 oz/125 g) unsweetened applesauce
1 cup (8 oz/250 g) low-fat fruit-flavored yogurt
Decaffeinated coffee

Lunch

BBQ beef sandwich: 2 ounces (60 g) thin-sliced roast beef, topped with 1 tablespoon BBQ sauce, on a toasted onion roll
1 small ear of corn or ½ cup (3 oz/90 g) corn kernels
Mixed greens
2 tablespoons light cucumber dressing
1 fresh peach
1 cup (8 fl oz/250 mL) fat-free milk

Dinner

Honey Chicken on Apricot Wild Rice (see recipe on page 199)
Steamed asparagus (4 to 6 spears)
1 country-style biscuit
1 teaspoon soft margarine
½ tomato, sliced with fresh cilantro
½ cup (2 oz/60 g) mixed fresh berries
Hot herbal tea

Snack (anytime)

1 muffin
¾ cup (6 fl oz/180 mL) orange juice

Food servings — *Grains* 8; *Fruits* 4; *Vegetables* 5; *Dairy products* 2; *Poultry, seafood, meat* 2; *Legumes and nuts* 0; *Fats* 2; *Sweets* 0

Nutritional analysis — *Calories* 2,039; *Fat* 40 g; *Saturated fat* 16 g; *Cholesterol* 170 mg; *Sodium* 2,183 mg; *Fiber* 31 g

To further reduce sodium, top the roast beef sandwich with slices of fresh tomato and onion instead of BBQ sauce.

Menu-planning tip

By removing the skin from the chicken as called for in the recipe for Honey Chicken on Apricot Wild Rice, you save 50 calories and about 5 grams of fat.

Day 2

Breakfast

1 cup (1½ oz/45 g) bran cereal, topped with ½ cup (3 oz/90 g) dried mixed fruit (apples, apricots, raisins)
2 slices whole-grain toast
1 teaspoon soft margarine
1 cup (8 fl oz/250 mL) fat-free milk

Lunch

Turkey sandwich a la Mediterranean: ¼ cup (1 oz./30 g) cooked turkey, topped with 1 ounce (30 g) part-skim mozzarella cheese, ½ sliced tomato and 2 tablespoons commercially available pesto sauce, on two slices whole-wheat bread
1 kiwi
Mixed greens tossed with vinegar to taste and 1 teaspoon olive oil
¾ cup (6 fl oz/180 mL) unsalted vegetable juice

Dinner

Poached Salmon With Melon Salsa (see recipe on page 200)
Roasted red-skinned potatoes (3 small)
1 whole-wheat roll
1 tablespoon honey
1 cup (8 fl oz/250 mL) fat-free milk

Snack (anytime)

1 apple
⅓ cup (1 oz/30 g) unsalted nuts
¼ cup (½ oz/15 g) unsalted pretzels

Food servings — *Grains* 8; *Fruits* 4; *Vegetables* 4; *Dairy products* 3; *Poultry, seafood, meat* 1½ ; *Legumes and nuts* 1; *Fats* 3; *Sweets* 1

Nutritional analysis — *Calories* 2,010; *Fat* 62 g; *Saturated fat* 12 g; *Cholesterol* 112 mg; *Sodium* 1,725 mg; *Fiber* 30 g

To further reduce sodium, substitute fresh basil, a dash of olive oil and cracked black pepper on the turkey sandwich in place of pesto sauce.

Menu-planning tip

One kiwi provides 74 milligrams of vitamin C, all of your day's recommendation for vitamin C.

Day 3

Breakfast

1 cup (6 oz/185 g) fresh mixed fruits (melons, banana, apple, berries), topped with 1 cup (8 oz/250 g) low-fat vanilla-flavored yogurt and ⅓ cup (1 oz/30 g) toasted almonds
1 bran muffin
1 cup (8 fl oz/250 mL) fat-free milk
Herbal tea

Lunch

Curried chicken wrap: 1 medium flour tortilla filled with mixture of ⅓ cup (2 oz/60 g) cooked chopped chicken, ½ chopped apple, 2 tablespoons fat-free mayonnaise and ½ teaspoon curry powder
1 cup (4 oz/125 g) raw baby carrots
2 reduced-sodium rye crackers
1 nectarine
1 cup (8 fl oz/250 mL) fat-free milk

Dinner

Basil and Sun-Dried Tomato Fettuccine (see recipe on page 201)
Mixed greens
2 tablespoons low-fat Caesar dressing
1 whole-wheat roll
1 teaspoon margarine
Sparkling water

Snack (anytime)

Trail mix made with 2 tablespoons raisins, 3⁄4 cup (11⁄2 oz/45 g) unsalted minipretzels and 1⁄3 cup (1 oz/30 g) unsalted nuts

Food servings — *Grains* 7; *Fruits* 5; *Vegetables* 4; *Dairy products* 3; *Poultry, seafood, meat* 1; *Legumes and nuts* 2; *Fats* 2; *Sweets* 1
Nutritional analysis — *Calories* 2,109; *Fat* 59 g; *Saturated fat* 8 g; *Cholesterol* 61 mg; *Sodium* 1,310 mg; *Fiber* 30 g

Menu-planning tip

Eating more meals that don't include meat, such as this evening's Basil and Sun-Dried Tomato Fettuccine, can help lower both your blood pressure and your blood cholesterol. People who follow plant-based diets tend to have a lower risks for high blood pressure and heart disease.

Day 4

Breakfast

1 whole-wheat bagel
2 tablespoons peanut butter
1 medium orange
1 cup (8 fl oz/250 mL) fat-free milk
Decaffeinated coffee

Lunch

Spinach salad: Fresh spinach leaves mixed with 1 sliced pear, ½ cup (3 oz/90 g) mandarin orange sections, ⅓ cup (1 oz/30 g) unsalted peanuts and 2 tablespoons fat-free red wine vinaigrette
12 reduced-sodium wheat crackers
1 cup (8 fl oz/250 mL) fat-free milk

Dinner

Sweet Potato and Shrimp Gumbo (see recipe on page 202)
1 sourdough roll
1 teaspoon soft margarine
1 cup (4 oz/125 g) fresh berries with chopped mint
Herbal iced tea

Snack (anytime)

1 cup (8 oz/250 g) fat-free yogurt
8 vanilla wafers

Food servings — *Grains* 7; *Fruits* 5; *Vegetables* 4; *Dairy products* 3; *Poultry, seafood, meat* 1; *Legumes and nuts* 2; *Fats* 1; *Sweets* 0
Nutritional analysis — *Calories* 1,997; *Fat* 55 g; *Saturated fat* 7 g; *Cholesterol* 78 mg; *Sodium* 1,523 mg; *Fiber* 32 g

Menu-planning tip

Adding a pear and mandarin oranges to your spinach salad is an easy way to include more fruit in your diet. When combined with a glass of orange juice for breakfast, you've already tallied three fruit servings by lunch. These fruits also contain moderate to high amounts of potassium.

Day 5

Breakfast

1 cup (6 oz/185 g) cooked old-fashioned oatmeal, topped with 1 tablespoon brown sugar
2 slices whole-wheat toast
1 teaspoon soft margarine
1 banana
1 cup (8 fl oz/250 mL) fat-free milk

Lunch

Tuna salad: ½ cup (5 oz/155 g) drained, unsalted water-packed tuna, mixed with 2 tablespoons fat-free mayonnaise, 15 grapes and ¼ cup (1 oz./30 g) diced celery, served on romaine lettuce
12 low-sodium wheat crackers
1 cup (8 fl oz/250 mL) fat-free milk

Dinner

Teriyaki Vegetable and Beef Kabobs (see recipe on page 203)
1 cup (6 oz/180 g) steamed rice with parsley
⅛ (or 2 rings) pineapple
Green tea

Snack (anytime)

1 cup (8 oz/250 g) low-fat yogurt
1 banana

Food servings — *Grains* 8; *Fruits* 4; *Vegetables* 4; *Dairy products* 3; *Poultry, seafood, meat* 2; *Legumes and nuts* 0; *Fats* 2; *Sweets* 1
Nutritional analysis — *Calories* 2,010; *Fat* 40 g; *Saturated fat* 6 g; *Cholesterol* 190 mg; *Sodium* 1,950 mg; *Fiber* 33 g

To further reduce sodium, don't add salt when cooking the oatmeal.

Menu-planning tip

A simple way to ensure three servings of dairy foods is to include an 8-ounce glass of fat-free milk with each meal. Or as in today's menu, substitute low-fat yogurt for an equal amount of calcium. Dairy products are rich in calcium — a mineral that can help control blood pressure and keep your bones and teeth strong.

Day 6

Breakfast

1 English muffin
2 tablespoons fat-free cream cheese
1 cup (4 oz/125 g) fresh strawberries
1 cup (8 fl oz/250 mL) fat-free milk

Lunch

Lemon peppered chicken breast on rye: ½ grilled boneless chicken breast seasoned with lemon pepper, topped with shredded lettuce and 1 tablespoon low-fat mayonnaise, on two slices rye bread
1 cup (4 oz/125 g) fresh vegetables (raw baby carrots, celery sticks, broccoli florets)
2 reduced-sodium rye crackers
¾ cup (6 fl oz/180 mL) cranberry juice

Dinner

Rosemary Lamb and White Beans (see recipe on page 204)
1 cup (6 oz/180 g) steamed broccoli florets
1 slice whole-wheat bread
1 teaspoon soft margarine
1 fresh sliced pear sprinkled with balsamic vinegar
1 cup (8 fl oz/250 mL) fat-free milk

Snack (anytime)

1 cup (8 oz/250 g) low-fat cottage cheese
2 fresh apricots
4 graham crackers

Food servings — *Grains* 8; *Fruits* 4; *Vegetables* 4; *Dairy products* 3; *Poultry, seafood, meat* 2; *Legumes and nuts* 2; *Fats* 3; *Sweets* 0
Nutritional analysis — *Calories* 1,902; *Fat* 35 g; *Saturated fat* 4 g; *Cholesterol* 165 mg; *Sodium* 2,365 mg; *Fiber* 33 g

Using fresh instead of canned vegetables in the dinner recipe will further reduce sodium.

Menu-planning tip

The white beans in this evening's meal provide two servings of legumes — half your weekly goal. Beans are low fat and cholesterol-free. They also supply fiber, protein, potassium, calcium and magnesium.

Day 7

Breakfast

Southwestern omelet: 1 egg + 2 egg whites, 1½ ounces (45 g) low-fat cheddar cheese, ¼ cup (1 oz/30 g) chopped green or red bell peppers, ¼ cup (1½ oz/45 g) chopped tomato
1 medium cornmeal muffin
2 teaspoons fruit spread
¾ cup (6 fl oz/180 mL) orange juice
Decaffeinated coffee

Lunch

Vegetable pita: 1 whole-wheat pita stuffed with shredded lettuce, ½ of a medium-sized tomato, chopped, ¼ cucumber, sliced, ⅓ cup (1½ oz/45 g) feta cheese and 2 tablespoons light French dressing
10 cherries
1 cup (8 oz/250 g) frozen yogurt
Herbal tea

Dinner

Cruciferous Stir-Fry Over Rice (see recipe on page 205)
1 slice crusty bread
1 teaspoon soft margarine
1 fresh peach sprinkled with cinnamon
1 cup (8 fl oz/250 mL) fat-free milk

Snack (anytime)

2 cups (1 oz/30 g) unsalted air-popped popcorn
¾ cup (6 fl oz/180 mL) cranberry juice

Food servings — *Grains* 8; *Fruits* 4; *Vegetables* 5; *Dairy products* 3; *Poultry, seafood, meat* 1; *Legumes and nuts* 1; *Fats* 3; *Sweets* 1
Nutritional analysis — *Calories* 1,957; *Fat* 52 g; *Saturated fat* 19 g; *Cholesterol* 297 mg; *Sodium* 2,209 mg; *Fiber* 25 g

To further reduce sodium, look for low-sodium cheddar cheese.

Menu-planning tip
This evening's Cruciferous Stir-Fry Over Rice includes seasonings from the Orient. Orange zest, five-spice powder, ginger, garlic and zesty red pepper flakes eliminate the need for salty soy sauce.

Honey Chicken on Apricot Wild Rice

Honey Chicken

Serves: 6 — Preparation: 10 minutes — Cooking: 40 minutes

- 3 tablespoons wheat germ
- 2 tablespoons honey
- 1 tablespoon Dijon mustard
- 1 tablespoon canned apricot nectar or apricot jam
- ¾ teaspoon reduced-sodium soy sauce
- 6 skinless, bone-in chicken breast halves, 5 oz (155 g) each, trimmed of visible fat

Preheat an oven to 375 F (190 C).

In a small bowl, mix together the wheat germ, honey, mustard, apricot nectar or jam and soy sauce until well blended.

Arrange the chicken pieces, bone side down, on a baking sheet. Spread the wheat germ mixture evenly over the chicken breasts. Bake until the chicken is opaque throughout and the wheat germ mixture has formed a crust, 35 to 40 minutes.

To serve, divide the rice among individual plates. Top each with a chicken breast half.

Per serving — *Calories* 411; *Protein* 36 g; *Carbohydrates* 63 g; *Fat* 2 g; *Saturated fat* <1 g; *Cholesterol* 63 mg; *Sodium* 163 mg; *Fiber* 5 g

Apricot Wild Rice

Makes: 6 cups (2 pounds/1 kg) — Preparation: 20 minutes — Cooking: 1 hour

- 1 oz (30 g) dried shiitake mushrooms, stemmed
- 1½ cups (12 fl. oz./375 mL) warm water
- 2 cups (12 oz/375 g) wild rice, rinsed in a fine-mesh sieve under cold running water
- ½ cup (3 oz/90 g) coarsely chopped dried apricots
- 2 shallots, minced

In a small bowl, soak the mushrooms in the warm water until barely softened, about 20 minutes. Remove the mushrooms, reserving the liquid. Coarsely chop the mushrooms. Strain the mushroom-soaking liquid through a fine-mesh sieve into a measuring cup. Add enough water to equal 5 cups (40 fl oz/1.25 L) liquid. Pour the liquid into a large saucepan and bring to a boil. Add the wild rice, mushrooms, apricots and shallots. Return to a boil, cover and reduce heat to low. Cool until the rice is tender and all the liquid has been absorbed, 45 minutes to 1 hour.

Per serving — *Calories* 252; *Protein* 9 g; *Carbohydrates* 55 g; *Fat* <1 g; *Saturated fat* <1 g; *Cholesterol* 0 mg; *Sodium* 6 mg; *Fiber* 5 g

Poached Salmon With Melon Salsa

Poached Salmon

Serves: 6 — Preparation: 40 minutes — Cooking: 15 minutes

2 green (spring) onions, thinly sliced, including green portions
1½ teaspoons chopped fresh mint
1 teaspoon grated fresh ginger
3 tablespoons grated lime zest
1½ pounds (750 g) salmon fillets, skinned and cut into 6 pieces

Preheat an oven to 450 F (230 C).

In a small bowl, toss together the onions, mint, ginger and lime zest.

Place 6 pieces of aluminum foil, each 10 inches (25 cm) square, onto a work surface. Place a piece of salmon in the center of each square. Top each with an equal amount of the onion mixture. Fold in the edges of the foil and crimp to seal. Place the packets in a single layer on a baking sheet and bake until opaque throughout, 12 to 15 minutes.

Melon Salsa

1 honeydew melon, about 3 pounds (1.5 kg), peeled, seeded and cut into ½-inch (12-mm) cubes
1 yellow bell pepper (capsicum), seeded, stemmed and cut into ½-inch (12-mm) squares
¼ cup (2 fl oz/60 mL) lime juice
½ red (Spanish) onion, chopped
1 jalapeno chile, minced
2 tablespoons chopped fresh mint

Prepare the salsa while the salmon is baking. In a medium bowl, toss together the melon, pepper, lime juice, onion, jalapeno and mint.

To serve, transfer the contents of each salmon packet onto an individual plate. Top each with an equal amount of the salsa.

Per serving — *Calories* 261; *Protein* 24 g; *Carbohydrates* 14 g; *Fat* 12 g; *Saturated fat* 2 g; *Cholesterol* 67 mg; *Sodium* 83 mg; *Fiber* 2 g

Basil and Sun-Dried Tomato Fettuccine

Serves: 6 — Preparation: 15 minutes — Cooking: 15 minutes

⅓ cup (3 fl oz/80 mL) canned vegetable broth
⅓ cup (3 fl oz/80 mL) water
6 sun-dried tomatoes (not oil-packed), cut into thin strips
2 teaspoons olive oil
2 garlic cloves, crushed with a garlic press
¼ teaspoon red pepper flakes
12 oz (375 g) dried fettuccine or linguine
½ cup (¾ oz/20 g) lightly packed torn basil leaves
2 tablespoons grated Parmesan cheese
1 tablespoon dried bread crumbs

In a small saucepan over medium heat, bring the vegetable broth, water, sun-dried tomatoes, olive oil, garlic and red pepper flakes to a boil. Remove from heat, cover and keep warm.

Fill a large pot three-quarters full of water and bring to a boil. Add the pasta and cook until al dente, about 10 minutes, or according to package directions. Remove ¼ cup (2 fl oz/60 mL) of the cooking water, then drain the pasta thoroughly.

In a warmed serving bowl, combine the pasta, broth mixture, basil and reserved cooking water. Toss to combine and coat the pasta evenly with the sauce.

To make dried bread crumbs, choose a loaf of whole-wheat bread with a firm, course-textured crumb. If you want a finer consistency to the crumbs, trim away the crusts. With your hands, crumble the bread into a blender or food processor. Pulse the machine on and off until the crumbs reach the desired consistency. If you like drier crumbs for a crunchier consistency, spread them in a baking dish or on a baking sheet and put them in an oven set at its lowest temperature. Bake for about 1 hour, stirring occasionally, or until they feel thoroughly dry to the touch.

To serve, divide among individual plates. Top each with an equal amount of the Parmesan and bread crumbs.

Per serving — *Calories* 247; *Protein* 9 g; *Carbohydrates* 45 g; *Fat* 3 g; *Saturated fat* <1 g; *Cholesterol* 1 mg; *Sodium* 103 mg; *Fiber* 2 g

Sweet Potato and Shrimp Gumbo

Serves: 6 — Preparation: 25 minutes — Cooking: 30 minutes

¾ cup (6 fl oz/180 mL) tomato juice
1 onion, chopped
1 green bell pepper (capsicum), stemmed, seeded and chopped
½ pound (250 g) okra, stemmed and thinly sliced
2 celery stalks, chopped
⅔ cup (5 fl oz/160 mL) dry white wine
¼ cup (2 fl oz/60 mL) distilled white vinegar
1 pound (500 g) sweet potatoes, peeled and cut into 1-inch (2.5-cm) cubes
3 cups (28 oz/875 g) canned crushed tomatoes or tomato puree
1½ tablespoons chili powder
⅛ teaspoon cayenne pepper
24 fresh or thawed frozen shrimp (prawns), shelled and deveined
6 cups (32 oz/1 kg) cooked, hot white rice

In a large frying pan over medium-high heat, heat the tomato juice. Add the onion, bell pepper, okra and celery and saute until wilted and softened slightly, 5 to 7 minutes.

Add the wine and vinegar and bring to a boil. Stir in the sweet potatoes, tomatoes or puree, chili powder and cayenne and cook until it returns to a boil. Reduce heat to low, cover and simmer, stirring occasionally, until the sweet potatoes are tender, 15 to 18 minutes.

Add the shrimp and stir to combine. Cover and cook until the shrimp are pink, about 5 minutes.

To serve, divide the rice among individual bowls. Top each with an equal amount of the gumbo.

Per serving — *Calories* 362; *Protein* 14 g; *Carbohydrates* 72 g; *Fat* 2 g; *Saturated fat* <1 g; *Cholesterol* 49 mg; *Sodium* 397 mg; *Fiber* 6 g

Teriyaki Vegetable and Beef Kabobs

Serves: 6 — Preparation: 25 minutes — Marinating: 30 minutes — Cooking: 10 minutes

Marinade

½ cup (4 fl oz/125 mL) reduced-sodium soy sauce
4 garlic cloves, crushed with a garlic press
2 teaspoons grated fresh ginger
2 teaspoons lime juice
2 teaspoons honey
¼ teaspoon red pepper flakes
¼ teaspoon sesame oil

1 pound (500 g) beef tenderloin, trimmed of visible fat and cut into 1-inch (2.5-cm) cubes
3 Japanese eggplants (aubergines), cut crosswise into ½-inch (12-mm) pieces
1¼ pounds (625 g) white mushrooms
2 zucchini (courgettes), cut crosswise into ½-inch (12-mm) pieces
2 yellow squash, cut crosswise into ½-inch (12-mm) pieces
2 red bell peppers (capsicums), stemmed, seeded and cut into ¾-inch (2-cm) squares
2 red (Spanish) onions, cut into ½-inch-thick (12-mm) wedges

To make the marinade, in a large bowl, whisk together the soy sauce, garlic, ginger, lime juice, honey, pepper flakes and sesame oil. Transfer 3 tablespoons of the marinade to a medium bowl. Add the beef to the medium bowl, tossing to coat. Add the eggplants, mushrooms, zucchini, squash, peppers and onions to the large bowl, tossing to coat.

Cover and marinate both the meat and vegetables at room temperature for 30 minutes, tossing once or twice. (Note: If marinating longer than 30 minutes, place in refrigerator.)

Meanwhile, preheat a broiler (griller). Line the broiler pan with aluminum foil and coat with nonstick cooking spray. Soak 18 long wooden skewers in water to cover.

Using a slotted spoon, remove the meat and vegetables from the bowls and pat dry with paper towels. Discard the meat marinade.

For the 6 beef kabobs, divide the meat cubes equally among 6 skewers, threading it alternately with one-third of the mushrooms, zucchini, squash, peppers and onions.

For the 12 vegetable kabobs, thread the eggplant pieces onto 12 skewers, alternating with the remaining mushrooms, zucchini, squash, peppers and onions.

Working in batches if necessary, place the kabobs 2 inches (5 cm) apart on the broiler pan. Position the pan 4 inches (10 cm) from the heat source. Broil, turning once or twice and brushing the kabobs with any remaining vegetable marinade, until the vegetables are tender and the beef is nicely browned, 8 to 10 minutes.

To serve, place 1 beef and 2 vegetable kabobs on each plate.

Per vegetable kabob — *Calories* 35; *Protein* 2 g; *Carbohydrates* 7 g; *Fat* <1 g; *Saturated fat* 0 g; *Cholesterol* 0 mg; *Sodium* 181 mg; *Fiber* 1 g
Per beef kabob — *Calories* 160; *Protein* 18 g; *Carbohydrates* 8 g; *Fat* 6 g; *Saturated fat* 2 g; *Cholesterol* 48 mg; *Sodium* 393 mg; *Fiber* 1 g

Rosemary Lamb and White Beans

Serves: 6 — Preparation: 10 minutes — Marinating: 30 minutes — Cooking: 30 minutes

Rosemary Lamb

1½ teaspoons finely chopped fresh rosemary or ½ teaspoon dried rosemary
2 garlic cloves, crushed with a garlic press
½ teaspoon olive oil
6 loin lamb chops, 5 oz. (155 g) each, trimmed of visible fat

Beans

4½ cups (2 pounds/1 kg) cooked white beans or canned white beans, rinsed and drained
1½ cups (9 oz/280 g) diced fresh tomatoes or canned diced tomatoes, drained
1 small onion, finely chopped
½ cup (¾ oz/20 g) chopped fresh flat-leaf (Italian) parsley
1½ teaspoons chopped fresh rosemary or ½ teaspoon dried rosemary
3 garlic cloves, minced
¾ teaspoon ground pepper
6 small rosemary sprigs

In a small bowl, combine the rosemary, garlic and olive oil. Rub the mixture evenly into both sides of the lamb chops. Cover and marinate at room temperature for 30 minutes. (Note: If marinating longer than 30 minutes, place in refrigerator.)

For the beans, preheat an oven to 425 F (220 C). Coat a 2-quart (2-L) shallow baking dish with non-stick cooking spray.

In a large bowl, combine the beans, tomatoes, onion, parsley, rosemary, garlic and pepper.

Spread the bean mixture into the prepared dish. Cover and bake until heated through, about 15 minutes.

Meanwhile, preheat a broiler (griller). Arrange the lamb chops on a broiler pan and place the pan 4 inches (10 cm) from the heat. Broil, turning once, until lightly browned on both sides, 6 to 7 minutes total.

Remove the dish from the oven and arrange the lamb chops on top of the beans, pressing down gently. Return to the oven and cook, uncovered, until the beans are lightly browned on top and the chops are fully cooked, about 10 minutes.

To serve, divide the beans and lamb chops among individual plates. Garnish with the rosemary sprigs.

Per serving — *Calories* 354; *Protein* 32 g; *Carbohydrates* 43 g; *Fat* 7 g; *Saturated fat* 2 g; *Cholesterol* 51 mg; *Sodium* 61 mg; *Fiber* 7 g

Cruciferous Stir-Fry Over Rice

Serves: 6 — Preparation: 20 minutes — Cooking: 20 minutes

3½ cups (28 fl oz/875 mL) water
1 cup (8 fl oz/250 mL) canned vegetable broth
2 tablespoons grated orange zest
1½ teaspoons five-spice powder
3 cups (21 oz/655 g) basmati or Texmati rice
1 tablespoon canola oil
1 tablespoon minced fresh ginger
3 garlic cloves, minced
4 green (spring) onions, finely chopped, including green portions
¼ teaspoon red pepper flakes
1 pound (500 g) broccoli, cut into florets
1 pound (500 g) cauliflower, cut into florets
8 oz (250 g) firm tofu, drained, blotted dry and cut into ½-inch (12-mm) cubes
8 oz (250 g) oyster mushrooms, halved
1 tablespoon sesame seeds
1 tablespoon reduced-sodium soy sauce

In a large, heavy saucepan, bring the water, broth, orange zest and five-spice powder to a boil. Stir in the rice. When the liquid returns to a boil, cover and reduce heat to low. Simmer until the rice is tender and the liquid has been absorbed, about 18 minutes.

Remove the pan from heat and let stand 5 minutes, covered, then fluff the rice with a fork.

Meanwhile, in a wok or large nonstick frying pan over high heat, heat half the oil. Add half each of the ginger, garlic, green onions and pepper flakes, and stir-fry until fragrant, about 30 seconds. Add half the broccoli and cauliflower and stir-fry until the broccoli turns bright green, about 2 minutes.

Add half the tofu, mushrooms, sesame seeds and soy sauce, and stir-fry until the tofu is heated through and the vegetables are tender and crisp, 2 to 3 minutes. Transfer the mixture to a large bowl and keep warm. Repeat with the remaining ingredients.

To serve, divide the rice among individual plates. Top each with an equal amount of the vegetables and tofu.

Per serving — *Calories* 480; *Protein* 22 g; *Carbohydrates* 91 g; *Fat* 9 g; *Saturated fat* <1 g; *Cholesterol* 0 mg; *Sodium* 352 mg; *Fiber* 6 g

The recipes on pages 199 to 205 are used with permission from *The Mayo Clinic / Williams-Sonoma Cookbook*. Weldon Owen Inc., 1998.

Additional resources

Contact these organizations for more information about high blood pressure and associated conditions.

American Diabetes Association
1701 N. Beauregard St.
Alexandria, VA 22311
800-342-2383
www.diabetes.org

American Heart Association
7272 Greenville Ave.
Dallas, TX 75231
800-242-8721
www.americanheart.org

American Society of Hypertension
515 Madison Ave., Suite 1212
New York, NY 10022
212-696-9099
www.ash-us.org

Mayo Clinic Health Information
www.MayoClinic.com

National Heart, Lung, and Blood Institute
P.O. Box 30105
Bethesda, MD 20824-0105
Recorded information:
800-575-9355
www.nhlbi.nih.gov

National Hypertension Association
324 East 30th St.
New York, NY 10016
212-889-3557
www.nathypertension.org

National Institute of Diabetes and Digestive and Kidney Diseases
Office of Communications and Public Liaison
NIDDK, National Institute of Health
31 Center Drive, MSC 2560
Bethesda, MD 20892-2560
800-438-5383
www.niddk.nih.gov

National Kidney Foundation
30 East 33rd St., Suite 1100
New York, NY 10016
800-622-9010
www.kidney.org

National Stroke Association
9707 E. Easter Lane
Englewood, CO 80112
800-787-6537
www.stroke.org

Index

E

F

G

H

I

N